Treatment Approaches with
Suicidal Adolescents

An Einstein Psychiatry Publication

Publication Series of the Department of Psychiatry
Albert Einstein College of Medicine of Yeshiva University
New York, NY

Editor-in-Chief   Herman M. van Praag, M.D., Ph.D.
Associate Editor   Demitri Papolos, M.D.

Treatment Approaches with Suicidal Adolescents

Edited by

JAMES K. ZIMMERMAN
GREGORY M. ASNIS

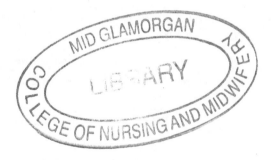

A Wiley-Interscience Publication

John Wiley & Sons, Inc.

New York • Chichester • Brisbane • Toronto • Singapore

This publication is designed to provide accurate and authoritative
information in regard to the subject matter covered. It is sold
with the understanding that the publisher is not engaged in
rendering professional services. If legal, accounting, medical,
psychological, or any other expert assistance is required, the
services of a competent professional person should be sought.

Library of Congress Cataloging-in-Publication Data:

Treatment approaches with suicidal adolescents / James K. Zimmerman,
   Gregory M. Asnis, editors.
      p.   cm. — (Publication series of the Department of Psychiatry
  Albert Einstein College of Medicine of Yeshiva University ; 11)
    Includes index.
    ISBN 0-471-10236-9 (cloth : alk. paper)
    1. Teenagers—Suicidal behavior.   2. Adolescent psychotherapy.
  I. Zimmerman, James K., 1949-   .   II. Asnis, Gregory M.
  III. Series.
    [DNLM: 1. Suicide, Attempted—in adolescence. 2. Psychotherapy-
  -in adolescence. 3. Psychotherapy—methods. 4. Crisis
  Intervention. WS 463 T7835 1995]
  RJ506.S9T74   1995
  616.89'022—dc20
  DNLM/DLC
  for Library of Congress   94-30990

Printed in the United States of America

10 9 8 7 6 5 4 3 2 1

Contributors

Seth Aronson, Psy.D., Assistant Director of Child and Adolescent Psychiatry, Albert Einstein College of Medicine/Bronx Municipal Hospital Center, Bronx, New York

Gregory M. Asnis, M.D., Professor of Psychiatry, Albert Einstein College of Medicine/Montefiore Medical Center, Bronx, New York

Robert Catenaccio, M.D., Clinical Assistant Professor of Psychiatry, Albert Einstein College of Medicine/Jacobi Hospital, Bronx, New York

Everett Dulit, M.D., Ph.D., Associate Clinical Professor of Psychiatry, Albert Einstein College of Medicine/Montefiore Medical Center, Bronx, New York

Lawrence A. Dyche, A.C.S.W, Senior Psychosocial Faculty, Department of Family Medicine, Albert Einstein College of Medicine/Montefiore Medical Center, Bronx, New York

Daniel E. Grosz, M.D., Assistant Professor of Psychiatry, UCLA Neuropsychiatric Institute, Los Angeles, California

David A. Jobes, Ph.D., Associate Professor of Psychology, The Catholic University of America, Washington, D.C.

Jeffrey P. Kahn, M.D., Clinical Assistant Professor of Psychiatry, New York Hospital/Cornell Medical Center, New York, New York

Valerie A. La Sorsa, Psy.D., Clinical Instructor of Psychiatry, Albert Einstein College of Medicine/Montefiore Medical Center, Bronx, New York

Antoon A. Leenaars, Ph.D., C.Psych., Private Practice, Windsor, Ontario, Canada

David Lester, Ph.D., Professor of Psychology, Stockton State College, Pomona, New Jersey

Karen J. Prowda, M.D., Private Practice, Binghamton, New York

Saul Scheidlinger, Ph.D., Professor Emeritus, Department of Psychiatry, Albert Einstein College of Medicine/Bronx Municipal Hospital Center, Bronx, New York

Bruce J. Schwartz, M.D., Assistant Professor of Psychiatry, Albert Einstein College of Medicine/Montefiore Medical Center, Bronx, New York

Paul D. Trautman, M.D., Assistant Professor of Psychiatry, New York Hospital/Cornell Medical Center, New York, New York

Martha E. Woodard, Psy.D., Staff Psychologist, Primary Children's Medical Center, Murray, Utah

Luis H. Zayas, Ph.D., Assistant Clinical Professor, Department of Family Medicine, Albert Einstein College of Medicine/Montefiore Medical Center, Bronx, New York

James K. Zimmerman, Ph.D., Assistant Professor, Department of Psychiatry, Albert Einstein College of Medicine/Montefiore Medical Center, Bronx, New York

A Note on the Series

Psychiatry is in a state of flux. The excitement springs in part from internal changes, such as the development and official acceptance (at least in the U.S.A.) of an operationalized, multiaxial classification system of behavioral disorders (the DSM-IV), the increasing sophistication of methods to measure abnormal human behavior, and the impressive expansion of biological and psychological treatment modalities. Exciting developments are also taking place in fields relating to psychiatry; in molecular (brain) biology, genetics, brain imaging, drug development, epidemiology, experimental psychology, to mention only a few striking examples.

More generally speaking, psychiatry is moving, still relatively slowly, but irresistibly, from a more philosophical, contemplative orientation, to that of an empirical science. From the fifties on, biological psychiatry has been a major catalyst of that process. It provided the mother discipline with a third cornerstone, that is, neurobiology, the other two being psychology and medical sociology. In addition, it forced the profession into the direction of standardization of diagnoses and of assessment of abnormal behavior. Biological psychiatry provided psychiatry not only with a new basic science and with new treatment modalities, but also with the tools, the methodology, and the mentality to operate within the confines of an empirical science, the only framework in which a medical discipline can survive.

In other fields of psychiatry, too, one discerns a gradual trend toward scientification. Psychological treatment techniques are standardized and manuals have been developed to make these skills more easily transferable. Methods registering treatment outcome—traditionally used in the behavioral/cognitive field—are now more and more requested and, hence, developed for dynamic forms of psychotherapy as well. Social and community psychiatry, until the sixties more firmly rooted in humanitarian ideals and social awareness than in empirical studies, profited greatly from its liaison with the social sciences and the expansion of psychiatric epidemiology.

Let there be no misunderstanding. Empiricism does *not imply* that it is only the measurable that counts. Psychiatry would be mutilated if it would neglect that which cannot be captured by numbers. It *does imply* that what is measurable should be measured. Progress in psychiatry is dependent on ideas and on experiment. Their linkage is inseparable.

This series, published under the auspices of the Department of Psychiatry of the Albert Einstein College of Medicine, Montefiore Medical Center, is meant to keep track of important developments in our profession, to summarize what has been achieved in particular fields, and to bring together the viewpoints obtained from disparate vantage points—in short, to capture some of the ongoing excitement in modern psychiatry, both in its clinical and experimental dimensions. The Department of Psychiatry at Albert Einstein College of Medicine hosts the series, but naturally welcomes contributions from others.

Bernie Mazel originally generated the idea—an ambitious plan that we all felt was worthy of pursuit. The edifice of psychiatry is impressive, but still somewhat flawed in its foundations. May this series contribute to consolidation of its infrastructure.

HERMAN M. VAN PRAAG, M.D., PH.D.
Professor and Chairman
Academic Psychiatric Center
University of Limburg
Maastricht
The Netherlands

Foreword

Joseph Richman

Drs. Zimmerman and Asnis have done a masterful job in editing and contributing to this important addition to our understanding and treatment of suicidal adolescents. It was a pleasure to read *Treatment Approaches with Suicidal Adolescents;* it is comprehensive and thorough in its topics, diverse in its points of view, and yet contains a unity of its own.

The young represent our future and the future of civilization. The prevalence of youthful suicide—the incidence has tripled in recent years—raises the specter that ours may be an endangered future. We need a total program of treatment, intervention, and prevention, one that encompasses all of society, starting with the family, in addition to the individual. Suicide is a message, telling us that much more than the fate of the individual adolescent is at stake.

I have labored intensively in the study and treatment of suicidal people of all ages. While reading this book, I felt in the company of old friends who were presenting their knowledge and expertise in assessment and treatment in the emergency room, on the wards, and in the clinics. They covered the place of crisis intervention, individual, group, and family therapies, and their integration with medication and other physical treatments. These writers carried me back in spirit to the intense and rewarding experiences that initiated my enduring fascination with suicide and its almost infinite variations.

Diversity stood out even within the different modalities, ranging from dynamic and analytic psychotherapy, cognitive behavior treatment, intervention with psychotropic drugs, and much more. The reader may be greatly tempted to try out all of these methods. While that may be unrealistic, the importance of being familiar with these procedures is uncontestable. The lesson that emerges is the value of an integrated approach combined with the flexibility of the therapists. I carried on an imaginary dialogue with the authors, agreeing most of the time, disagreeing at others, but being stimulated throughout.

The unity behind the diversity becomes most evident in reviewing what the different authors say about the treatment process. In general, they emphasized the following features.

First, the presence of a positive doctor-patient relationship is needed.

Second, a positive emphasis is required. In Chapter 8, for example, Paul Trautman said the adolescent and family must leave the first session with "a list of their strengths—the things that *aren't* wrong."

Third, a comprehensive and integrated orientation is necessary. Chapter 9 on family therapy is subtitled "An Integrated Approach." In Chapter 8 Trautman lists "collaboration between therapist and family" as a primary characteristic of the treatment. Suicide is one aspect of the stream of human unhappiness in general and of psychiatric and emotional disturbances in particular. These issues have a great deal in common, but that does not explain why an adolescent turns to suicide rather than to some other resolution. That is where the integrative approach emphasized in this book is so valuable for both understanding and intervention.

Fourth, it must be realized that suicide is precipitated by a crisis. The crisis nature of the etiology and treatment of the suicidal adolescent is insufficiently attended to in the literature. The reader can only be thankful that crisis assessment and intervention is dealt with so well in this book.

Fifth, the clash between adolescent developmental demands and family roles and relationships must be understood. Intergenerational conflict in the etiology of a suicidal state in adolescence is universal, as Luis Zayas and Lawrence Dyche demonstrate in their description of attempted suicide in Puerto Rican females in Chapter 11. The details may differ in different cultural groups, but suicidal adolescents emerge as much more alike than different.

Sixth, it is important to recognize both unity and diversity. Suicidal people possess a great deal in common. Nevertheless, in order to be an effective psychotherapist, it is necessary to know and be sensitive to the unique cultural heritage and background, family styles and values, and other social conditions impinging upon the suicidal adolescent.

The book ends with the questions "Does it work?" and "Is it worth it?" Look at all the pain, stress, and the distressing countertransference turmoil that plague the therapist. I may add that these emotional reactions are found especially in those beginning therapists who are the most empathic and promising. My response, which is implicit throughout this book, is that working with the suicidal adolescent is a uniquely worthwhile, rewarding task, and an invaluable growth and learning experience for the therapist.

But that does not mean it is easy. To paraphrase what Gerald Zuk said about family therapy, "If you can't stand the heat of treating the suicidal, get out of the kitchen." But if you get out, you may never become a good cook—or therapist. This book will help you become one.

Preface

An increase in suicidal behavior among adolescents has been a significant social problem over the past 40 years in the United States, with completed suicide having tripled in incidence between the 1950s and the 1980s. Estimates are that approximately 5,000 adolescents commit suicide each year, and that there may be 50 to 100 times as many who make suicide attempts. Further, suicide attempters are at much higher risk of eventual completed suicide than are nonattempters. Despite the relative rarity of adolescent suicide—there are 11 to 13 such deaths annually per 100,000 individuals age 15 to 24—its impact in human suffering is far greater, both in the toll on the lives of those directly associated with the suicide and on the psyche of society at large.

Faced with this devastating problem, a fairly large body of literature has developed concerning the profiles of adolescent suicide attempters and completers, including a focus on biological, psychosocial, ethnic, and familial risk factors. Likewise, the areas of assessment and prediction have received considerable attention in recent years. However, effective prevention and treatment techniques with suicide attempters are less well understood.

This volume focuses centrally on the assessment and treatment of adolescent suicide attempters, with the assumption that advances in the identification and treatment of this population will reduce the risk of future completed suicides among teens. The volume is both timely and significant in that its central concern is to offer specific and practical technical approaches with this high-risk population. All authors are seasoned clinicians—and many experienced researchers as well—who have devoted considerable professional time and energy to providing direct mental health services to suicidal adolescents.

The audience for this volume is wide, and includes mental health practitioners with various training backgrounds—such as psychiatrists, psychologists, social workers, nurses, crisis intervention workers—and staff of numerous facilities that have contact with troubled adolescents (including schools and other agencies in the community). Our intent is that these practitioners will gain further understanding of the specifics of treatment approaches, including the presentation of case examples, which in turn may have immediate ameliorative impact on their professional contacts with adolescents.

The overall structure of this book is designed to parallel the experience of working with suicidal adolescents from initial exposure through follow-up, in the following sequence: (1) an understanding of risk factors, diagnosis, and assessment; (2) the management of initial contact; (3) crisis intervention; (4) implementation of treatment in various modalities; and (5) long-term follow-up as an evaluative and therapeutic intervention.

To this end, Chapter 1 provides an introduction to work with suicidal adolescents from a clinical perspective, including the difficulties of this work along with its rewards, while Chapter 2 provides the reader with an understanding of current thinking regarding risk and protective factors in adolescent suicide.

Chapters 3 through 6 focus attention on the first phases of contact, including the assessment of suicidality in adolescents, treatment within the contexts of the emergency room and brief inpatient hospitalization, and a method for increasing initial compliance with treatment through the provision of a multifamily psychoeducational intake group.

Chapters 7 through 13 present various approaches to treatment. Each chapter that presents a treatment approach also employs case material to illustrate different approaches to treatment dictated by various symptom presentations. The first two of these chapters focus on the individual, in both psychodynamic (Chapter 7) and cognitive-behavioral (Chapter 8) treatment modalities. Chapter 9 presents a treatment approach that uses the family as the medium for therapeutic leverage, and Chapter 10 considers issues in group treatment with adolescent suicide attempters. Given the fact that past research suggests that there may be specific issues regarding treatment with Hispanic adolescent suicide attempters, Chapter 11 concerns this ethnic population. Chapter 12 presents issues in the psychopharmacological treatment of adolescent suicide attempters as well as the implications of various symptom presentations for decisions regarding medication regimens. Chapter 13 investigates the issue of long-term follow-up and the use of such follow-up as a therapeutic intervention and as a method to reduce recidivism. Finally, Chapter 14 provides a summary of the volume, including some reflections on the value and efficacy of treatment with suicidal adolescents along with some comments on the selection of approaches to such treatment.

In sum, the intent of this volume is to provide a guide to treatment approaches with suicidal adolescents, taking into account current knowledge in the field regarding assessment and biological, psychological, and social risk factors. It is hoped that the volume will be found directly useful clinically for practitioners; moreover, it also is meant to be interesting and stimulating for those who are more involved in theoretical and research issues with suicidal adolescents.

JAMES K. ZIMMERMAN, PH.D.
GREGORY M. ASNIS, M.D.

Acknowledgments

In conceptualizing and bringing to fruition a project such as the production of an edited volume, the support of numerous individuals is necessary. In this light, the authors would like to acknowledge a debt of gratitude to Herman M. van Praag, M.D., Ph.D., who was instrumental in fostering the birth of this volume, and to the Editorial Board of the Albert Einstein College of Medicine Monograph Series for their comments and critiques of the proposal for the book. We also would like to express our appreciation for the involvement and support of Herb Reich, of John Wiley & Sons, Inc., whose even-tempered, informal, and forthright approach to his work has been inspirational in nurturing the project through the vicissitudes of editorship and publication. Further, we would like to acknowledge the participation of Daniel E. Grosz, M.D., in the early phases of preparation.

In addition, and respectfully, we would like to acknowledge the involvement and cooperation of the authors who produced chapters for the volume. At times, they had to wait for feedback and comments for several months; at other times, they were expected to return revisions to us within days of their receipt of our comments. For the most part, their forebearance and good nature were impressive, and are deeply appreciated.

Finally, the first author would like to thank his wife, Jan Braun, publicly for the (nearly) constant support she showed over the long stretch required for the production of this book and for her consistent faith in his talents and abilities.

Contents

PART I
Introduction

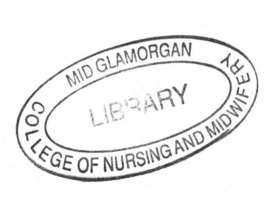

1

Treating Suicidal Adolescents
Is It Really Worth It?

JAMES K. ZIMMERMAN

It is unfortunate, but perhaps at this time axiomatic, to say that adolescent suicide is a major psychosocial problem. In the United States, recent studies suggest that between 5 and 10 percent of adolescents have made suicide attempts (Gallup, 1991, 1994; Harkavy Friedman, Asnis, Boeck, & DiFiore, 1987; Smith & Crawford, 1986), while 12 to 15 percent have "come close" and approximately 60 percent know of a peer who has attempted suicide (Gallup, 1991, 1994). Other studies have indicated that over 60 percent of adolescents also have had suicidal ideation at some time in their lives (Harkavy Friedman et al., 1987; Smith & Crawford, 1986; Zimmerman & Morledge, 1992). Suicide is currently the third leading cause of death among 15- to 24-year-olds, and, although its rate has stabilized in recent years, nearly 5,000 adolescents die by their own hand in the United States each year (National Center for Health Statistics, 1989, 1992). Moreover, this incidence increased threefold from the 1950s to the 1980s (Berman & Jobes, 1991; Fingerhut & Kleinman, 1988), and the rate may in fact be higher because it is likely that some suicides are officially reported as "accidents" or attributed to other causes (Berman & Jobes, 1991; Jobes & Berman, 1984).

It is estimated that there are 50 to 100 attempters for each completed adolescent suicide per year, leading to an annual attempter population of perhaps 250,000 to 500,000 individuals (Allen, 1987; Jacobziner, 1965). Further, it is clearly documented that a suicide attempt is one of the strongest risk factors for death by suicide (Farberow, 1989; Maris, 1981, 1992; Paarregaard, 1975; Shafii, Carrigan, Whittinghill, & Derrick, 1985); by making a suicide attempt, an adolescent's risk of eventual suicide increases tenfold (Lester, 1992).

3

DOES TREATMENT WORK?

Although a number of excellent volumes have been published on risk factors, assessment, prediction, and prevention of adolescent suicide, the magnitude of the problem remains daunting. In fact, in view of considerable urgency regarding a phenomenon that devastates not only by ending lives so prematurely but also by frequently destroying the lives of many others close to the adolescent who suicides, and despite the fact that numerous courageous clinicians and school personnel are engaged in intervention efforts, little is known about what approaches to intervention and treatment can be said *definitively* to prevent adolescent suicidality in the first place (primary prevention), to end a suicidal crisis once it has begun (secondary prevention), or to reduce recidivism once a suicide attempt has occurred (tertiary prevention). Recent studies indicate that treatment apparently does not reduce the likelihood that a youthful suicide attempter will repeat such behavior or even eventually die by suicide (Feiner, Adan, & Silverman, 1992; Pfeffer, Peskin, & Siefker, 1992; Pfeffer, Hurt, Kakuma, Peskin, Siefker, & Nagabhairava, 1994; Muehrer, 1990).

How should this information be integrated? How should practitioners who work with suicidal adolescents absorb the possibility that their efforts might be for naught? There are several answers to these questions, made not only in the service of resolving cognitive dissonance, but also based on clinical reality and knowledge derived from direct clinical experience. First of all, the fact that treatment approaches taken together—and viewed through the lens of statistical quantification—do not appear to reduce recidivism among suicidal adolescents does not mean categorically that treatment interventions are ineffective if not counterproductive. Studies to date have not specified what forms of treatment have been implemented, with what frequency over what period of time, in which setting, and with what theoretical perspectives and technical substrates. Simply put, controlled comparative treatment outcome studies have not been reported. Clearly, this is in part a result of the high-risk, crisis-oriented nature of work with suicidal adolescents and of the consequent ethical difficulties with prescribing a certain manualized treatment approach or relegating some individuals to no-treatment control groups.

Thus, quantitative studies may miss the subtleties of treatment success or failure by grouping together individuals who are in fact disparate in their likely responsiveness to psychotherapeutic intervention. The case study method has demonstrated that some suicidal adolescents do seem to respond well to some forms of treatment. A number of excellent articles and volumes have been written describing approaches to treatment with suicidal adolescents; many of these include case examples of successful treatment (e.g., Berman & Jobes, 1991; Fishman, 1988).

A second reason why treatment for suicidal adolescents does not appear to attenuate recidivism or reduce the likelihood of eventual suicide may be that this population is a deeply troubled one at the outset and chronically prone to continued emotional disturbance and psychosocial turmoil. The salient question in this regard is this: What would be the long-term prognosis for such individuals if they had no contact with mental health professionals and others in the community whose mission is to improve their lot, such that no treatment were implemented? Quite possibly their lives would be even more problematic, with an even higher likelihood that they would repeat suicidal behavior and complete suicide. A brief analogy from a more dire circumstance: If one is assessing the use of a new medication for cancer, one implements clinical trials with those who are already deemed terminally ill. Some who subsequently die were bound to die in any case; conversely, if even a few survive past their predicted span of life, the drug might prove to have some efficacy. In parallel, although treatment may not keep all suicidal adolescents from eventual death by suicide, intervention still may be effective in reducing continued suicidal behavior and in preventing some suicides.

EXPERIENCE IN THE TRENCHES

In light of this, the goals of treatment with suicidal adolescents, and the expectations of clinicians engaged in this treatment, must be considered carefully. They must be weighed against what we already know, which is that these individuals are at high risk for self-destructive behavior and may continue to be so for some time, even if treatment is effective in ameliorating their circumstances and reducing the intensity of their "unendurable psychic pain" (Maltsberger, 1986; Schneidman, 1985, 1988).

What, then, are challenges for the clinician engaged in interventions with suicidal adolescents? What are the likely reactions and countertransferences? What are the rewards? These questions will be considered in the next sections, followed by a few thoughts on what might be deemed successful treatment with this population.

Anxiety and Other Countertransference

When a clinician who works with suicidal adolescents tells others what he or she does professionally, the reaction is often "Oh, that must be extremely difficult work"; sometimes the response is simply a sigh and a look of commiseration. Frequently, after an uncomfortable pause, the conversation abruptly shifts to another topic unless the suicidologist persists. In fact, such clinicians are "in the trenches," "on the front lines," and frequently they have chosen to stay there. They stay there despite being constantly concerned that one patient or another may choose to end life prematurely; despite being aware that if a patient does so choose, actually very little can be done at that moment to prevent the suicide unless the adolescent is interrupted by chance or by his or her own ambivalence.

Invariably, clinicians treating suicidal adolescents must be able to experience, tolerate, and titrate large quantities of anxiety. There is the anxiety attendant upon interaction with individuals in crisis, and particularly the kind of crisis in which one of the acknowledged alternatives for regaining a form of control is self-destruction, a method that in many ways is out of the clinician's control. There is also the anxiety concomitant with concerns about the ethical issues involved in treating people where confidentiality may have to be broken, and where there are repeated questionings and self-doubts about when this line should or must be crossed. Further, perhaps more deep-seated anxieties are forced upon the clinician by persistent confrontation with his or her own existential issues regarding death and mortality. Work with suicidal adolescents compels one to ask what are the conditions under which one's own life might no longer feel worth living. Finally, there is the anxiety engendered by the upsurge of countertransference feelings in response to the adolescent's behavior; frequently these feelings include countertransference hate, so eloquently described by Maltsberger and Buie (1974) and often so intolerable for many clinicians.

In addition to anxiety, many clinicians experience moments, or even extended periods, of powerlessness, frustration, inefficacy, and doubt about their clinical skills while treating suicidal adolescents (e.g., see

Zimmerman, 1994). Sometimes these reactions are infused with the intensity of countertransference hate; other times they have the potential to impel such countertransference to develop. In either case, the clinician may find it difficult not to act out in the relationship with the patient, which can lead to undesirable and sometimes dangerous consequences, such as the patient's withdrawal from treatment or an upsurge in suicidality (Maltsberger & Buie, 1974).

Clearly, such reactions are engendered and fostered at least partially by the adolescent's current psychological state. Many, if not all, suicidal adolescents certainly are experiencing some form of self-hatred; many also are filled with anger expressed outward as well as against themselves. Many are provocative, controlling, rebellious, irresponsible, and often ungratifying to interact with. Nevertheless, it is also obvious that to respond to such provocations in anything but a controlled, mature, therapeutic way could convey to the adolescent that here is simply one more person who feels he or she does not belong among the living any longer. This is a pathway to stagnant, if not destructive, treatment.

The Positive Side

How do mental health professionals who treat suicidal adolescents manage this roiling of emotions without either acting out or giving up the work? Many use collegial support and peer supervision; some, in fact, regard this as an essential component of professional life if they are to stay "in the trenches" with patients who might kill themselves (Richman, 1986). Many also titrate their anxiety, frustration, and powerlessness through other means, such as gallows humor. Some move into other areas of clinical practice and carry only one or two suicidal adolescents in their caseload at any given time.

Those who are able to stay with this sometimes wrenching but always challenging work often have a somewhat paradoxical response when others commiserate on how difficult the work must be: They recognize the optimistic side and the potential for real and enduring change that can be accomplished within and because of a suicidal crisis involving an adolescent. In part, this is consequent to the fact that adolescents often are aware that, at least in some aspects, their suicidal behavior is an expression of the need and desire for change, a plea for transformation of an intolerable situation.

Mobilization

The suicidal crisis thus can become a rallying point, mobilizing the resources of the adolescent and family in ways that did not seem plausible in the past. In this respect, when suicidal adolescents and their families begin treatment, there is frequently a sense of desperation, a recognition that "something's got to be done," that does not exist within the enduring, often psychopathogenic quotidian experience that preceded the eruption of suicidal behavior. There is a potential for intensity of engagement and an urgent willingness to work, even if it sometimes does not feel that way to the treating clinician, who may be confronted more with apparent resistance, lack of commitment, or sabotage of the intervention. If the need for assistance can be grasped and pulled into the forefront so that layers of denial and superficial nonchalance do not encumber the treatment, some adolescents and their families clearly perceive the value of interventions offered by mental health professionals; consequently, impressive strides toward regaining emotional balance and attenuation of family dysfunction can be made. This work then can lead to a decrease in the adolescent's suicidality.

Problem Solving

Further, a suicide attempt in adolescence is often an expression of the effort to solve an "insolvable problem" (Orbach, 1986, 1988; Zimmerman, 1991, 1993a)—that is, a problem that apparently does not allow a solution which avoids a profound experience of loss, pain, or unacceptable compromise. In such a situation, the clinician can work with and support the adolescent's desire to find a solution, to be creative in ameliorating his or her life circumstances in ways that are less self-destructive. In a sense, one can say, "That was one way to change your lot; can you think of some others that don't hurt you so much?" Engaged in this perspective on the suicidal crisis, adolescents (and their families) again are often able to make perceptible progress in a fairly brief period of time. This seems to be the case particularly if the problem can be seen as one in which all concerned have a role, but in which no one is singled out for full blame. When this is true, the adolescent and available members of the family can understand the problem as one in which they are mutually enmired and from which they can extricate themselves together.

Case Example

At age 16, Tanya ingested a large overdose of various medications with intent to die after she felt betrayed and rejected by her mother, with whom she lived alone. She felt that her efforts to become more mature, including finding friends outside the home and becoming sexually active, were misunderstood by her mother, who insisted that Tanya stay at home at all times and cleave to more traditional social values, such as respect for her elders and sexual chastity before marriage. After the suicide attempt, Tanya felt that her mother was becoming even more intrusive; for her part, Tanya's mother felt "pushed around" and forced into a position of letting her daughter do "what she wanted to" rather than "what was right."

In treatment, the therapist helped them see the crisis in the context of the overarching issue of Tanya's development and movement toward adulthood. Both Tanya and her mother were then freer to examine their own roles and responsibilities in relation to this issue and to each other. They began to address more directly the arduous task of evolving toward a relationship of mother and adult daughter, and were more able to engage in this process as partners, as problem-solvers, rather than as adversaries.

Hopefulness

When faced with potential adolescent suicide, many people—often including the teen's parents—respond by saying "But he has his whole life ahead of him" or "She has so much to live for." It is indeed difficult, without some depth of examination, to comprehend why an individual would want to end his or her life so near to its outset. Nevertheless, obviously many adolescents do embark on a self-destructive trajectory, and they rarely want to hear how much they have to live for; in general, this simply does not help them feel more like living.

Ironically, then, given the hopelessness experienced by so many suicidal adolescents, some of the hopefulness that many mental health professionals experience in interaction with them is based on the above-mentioned concept: In essence, many clinicians and school personnel know that these individuals *do* have a lot to live for, that they *do* have their whole life ahead of them, that they have not yet really begun to discover the things of which they are capable. This is part of what makes work with suicidal adolescents worthwhile. The clinician can see the potential for the future if the adolescent gets on the right track, even if the adolescent cannot. Part of the challenge of intervention, then, is to instill some of this fragile, nascent (or dormant) hope in the adolescent.

Successful Treatment

In considering what constitutes successful treatment with suicidal adolescents, the most obvious answer is that suicidality must be attenuated and suicidal behavior prevented. Other symptoms must be addressed as well, through either psychotherapy or pharmacotherapy, or both. However, there are many avenues toward the goal of a decrease or cessation of suicidality, depending on the issues and circumstances presented in each case. Often, as issues resolve and circumstances improve, suicidality wanes.

One issue that frequently inheres in the etiology of adolescent suicidality is the inexorable engine of maturation and development, and its effects on the experience of the adolescent and his or her family (Rich, Kirkpatrick-Smith, Bonner, & Jans, 1992; Wade, 1987; Zimmerman, 1991, 1993a). In cases where this issue takes center stage, treatment is likely to require the participation of the family; if this is not possible, it may be necessary to support the adolescent in separating from the home. In any case, the goal here, and therefore the measure of success, is the resolution of the current developmental crisis so that the adolescent may resume more normative progress toward adulthood.

Another frequent etiological factor in adolescent suicide is the experience of loss and disconnection. A large percentage of suicide attempts in adolescence occur subsequent to an argument or break-up with a boy- or girlfriend or to a fight with parents (Barter, Swaback, & Todd, 1968; Pfeffer, 1989; Rotheram-Borus & Trautman, 1988; Shaffer, 1974; Simonds, McMahon, & Armstrong, 1991; Zimmerman, 1993a). Some authors suggest a diathesis in this regard as a result of early losses through parental death, divorce, or separation (Adam, 1981; Furst & Huffine, 1991; Holinger, 1989; Lester, 1992; Pfeffer, 1986, 1989; Slater & Depue, 1981). In such instances, then, successful treatment should be marked by an improvement in the adolescent's ability to experience loss without resorting to self-destructive action.

In fact, factors that promote connectedness, belongingness, and a sense of support apparently attenuate suicidality (Garmezy, 1985;

Maris, 1991; Pfeffer, 1989; Sanborn, 1990; Yufit, 1991). Adolescents who are suicidal often do not have solid and consistent support systems (King, Raskin, Gdowski, Butkus, & Opipari, 1990; Pfeffer, 1989), and therefore success in treatment also might be measured in some instances by an increase in supports and in the adolescent's ability to seek out, secure, and maintain supports in the home, school, and community.

In certain cases, academic difficulties, often with underlying learning disabilities, can contribute to an upsurge in suicidality (Rourke, 1988; Rourke, Young, & Leenaars, 1989; Shaffer, 1988; Shaffer, Garland, Gould, Fisher, & Trautman, 1988; Zimmerman, 1993b). Consequently, a direct focus on these issues, and their impact on the adolescent, family members, and school, can have an ameliorative effect. In this regard, treatment success could be indicated by the adolescent's ability to resume learning at his or her level of capability and by a reorienting of attitudes toward the adolescent's behavior, so that it is seen as sequelae of the disability and not as a result of stupidity, oppositionalism, or laxity in motivation (e.g., see Zimmerman, 1994). In the best scenario, this reorientation should occur within the adolescent, in the family, and in the educational setting as well.

In general, successful treatment often will include an increase in hopefulness in the adolescent (and perhaps also within the family), an improvement in problem-solving skills, and the development of a sense of balance, confidence, and efficacy. Finally, given that suicidality in adolescence often accompanies chronic issues and circumstances that do not lend themselves easily to ameliorative transformation, successful treatment may need to encompass an increased ability to tolerate psychic pain and unfortunate environments (both familial and geographic). Although some suicidal adolescents experience a cessation of most or all suicidal thought as well as behavior, some can be expected to improve only in their ability to experience suicidal ideation without feeling compelled to act on it.

CONCLUSION

In ending, it is salient to point out, as a cautionary note, that there are some cases that reach as satisfactory a conclusion as did that of Tanya and her mother. This is not to say that all, or even perhaps the majority, of treatment cases with suicidal adolescents are as heartening. In fact, suicidologists know that many adolescents are not very responsive to treatment, nor are their families; many others do not even avail them-selves of mental health services at any time (Clarke, 1988; Rotheram-Borus, 1990; Swedo, 1989; Trautman & Rotheram, 1986). Further, there are times when the adolescent may feel improved enough and sta-ble enough to end treatment, while the clinician is left thinking that the work is only half done.

Nevertheless, it is perhaps because of those individuals and families who do make impressive and enduring progress, deeply moving to the clinician fortunate enough to assist them, that some mental health pro-fessionals are able to continue their work with such a difficult, frus-trating, and gut-wrenching population. Sometimes it works, and works beautifully—and that may be the best answer when one is asked how one can tolerate working with suicidal adolescents.

REFERENCES

Adam, K. S. (1981). Parental loss and family disorganization in the predis-position to suicidal behavior. In J. P. Soubrier & J. Vedrinne (Eds.), *De-pression and suicide* (pp. 533–537). Paris, France: Pergamon Press.

Allen, B. (1987). Youth suicide. *Adolescence, 22,* 271–290.

Barter, J., Swaback, D., & Todd, D. (1968). Adolescent suicide attempts: A follow-up study of hospitalized patients. *Archives of General Psychi-atry, 19,* 523–527.

Berman, A. L., & Jobes, D. A. (1991). *Adolescent suicide: Assessment and intervention.* Washington, DC: American Psychological Association.

Clarke, C. F. (1988). Deliberate self-poisoning in adolescents. *Archives of Disorders of Childhood, 63,* 1479–1483.

Farberow, N. L. (1989). Preparatory and prior suicidal behaviors. In Alcohol, Drug Abuse, and Mental Health Administration, *Report of the Secre-tary's Task Force on Youth Suicide (vol. 2): Risk factors for youth suicide* (pp. 34–55). (DHHS Publication No. ADM 89-1622). Washington, DC: U.S. Government Printing Office.

Feiner, R. D., Adan, A. M., & Silverman, M. M. (1992). Risk assessment and prevention of youth suicide in schools and educational contexts. In R. W. Maris, A. L. Berman, J. T. Maltsberger, & R. I. Yufit (Eds.), *Assessment and prediction of suicide* (pp. 420–447). New York: The Guilford Press.

Fingerhut, L. A., & Kleinman, J. C. (1988). Letter to the editor, "Suicide Notes for Young People," *Journal of the American Medical Association, 259,* 356.

Fishman, H. C. (1988). *Treating troubled adolescents: A family therapy approach.* New York: Basic Books.

Furst, J., & Huffine, C. L. (1991). Assessing vulnerability to suicide. *Suicide and Life-Threatening Behavior, 21*(4), 329–344.

Gallup (1991). Teenage suicide study: Executive Summary, March 1991. Princeton, NJ: The Gallup Organization.

Gallup (1994). Teenage suicide study: Executive Summary, June 1994. Princeton, NJ: The Gallup Organization.

Garmezy, N. (1985). Stress-resistant children: The search for protective factors. In J. E. Stevenson (Ed.), Recent research in developmental psychopathology. *Journal of Child Psychology and Psychiatry Book Supplement* (No. 4, pp. 213–233). Oxford, UK: Pergamon Press.

Harkavy Friedman, J. M., Asnis, G. M., Boeck, M., & DiFiore, J. (1987). Prevalence of specific suicidal behaviors in a high school sample. *American Journal of Psychiatry, 144*(9), 1203–1206.

Holinger, P. C. (1989). Epidemiological issues in youth suicide. In C. R. Pfeffer (Ed.), *Suicide among youth: Perspectives on risk and prevention* (pp. 41–62). Washington, DC: American Psychiatric Press.

Jacobziner, H. (1965). Attempted suicide in adolescence. *Journal of the American Medical Association, 10,* 22–36.

Jobes, D. A., & Berman, A. L. (1984, October). *Response biases and the impact of psychological autopsies on medical examiners' determination of mode of death.* Paper presented at the 17th Annual Meeting of the American Association of Suicidology, Anchorage, AK.

King, C. A., Raskin, A., Gdowski, C. L., Butkus, M., & Opipari, L. (1990). Psychosocial factors associated with urban adolescent female suicide attempts. *Journal of the American Academy of Child and Adolescent Psychiatry, 29*(2), 289–294.

Lester, D. (1992). *Why people kill themselves* (3rd ed.). Springfield, IL: Charles C. Thomas.

Maltsberger, J. T. (1986). *Suicide risk: The formulation of clinical judgment.* New York: New York University Press.

Maltsberger, J. T., & Buie, D. H. (1974). Countertransference hate in the treatment of suicidal patients. *Archives of General Psychiatry, 30,* 625–633.

Maris, R. W. (1981). *Pathways to suicide.* Baltimore, MD: Johns Hopkins University Press.

Maris, R. W. (1991). Introduction to special issue: Assessment and prediction of suicide. *Suicide and Life-Threatening Behavior, 21*(1), 1–17.

Maris, R. W. (1992). The relationship of nonfatal suicide attempts to completed suicide. In R. W. Maris, A. L. Berman, J. T. Maltsberger, & R. I. Yufit (Eds.), *Assessment and prediction of suicide* (pp. 362–380). New York: The Guilford Press.

Muehrer, P. (1990). *Conceptual research models for preventing mental disorders* (DHHS Publications No. ADM 90-1713). Rockville, MD: National Institute of Mental Health.

National Center for Health Statistics. (1989). *Monthly vital statistics report* (vol. 37, no. 13). Hyattsville, MD: U.S. Public Health Service.

National Center for Health Statistics. (1992). *Monthly vital statistics report* (vol. 40, no. 8). Hyattsville, MD: U.S. Public Health Service.

Orbach, I. (1986). The "insolvable problem" as a determinant in the dynamics of suicidal behavior in children. *American Journal of Psychotherapy, 40*(4), 511–520.

Orbach, I. (1988). *Children who don't want to live*. San Francisco: Jossey-Bass.

Paarregaard, G. (1975). Suicide among attempted suicides: A 10-year follow-up. *Suicide and Life-Threatening Behavior, 5*(3), 140–144.

Pfeffer, C. R. (1986). *The suicidal child*. New York: The Guilford Press.

Pfeffer, C. R. (1989). Life stress and family risk factors for youth fatal and nonfatal suicidal behavior. In C. R. Pfeffer (Ed.), *Suicide among youth: Perspectives on risk and prevention* (pp. 143–164). Washington, DC: American Psychiatric Press.

Pfeffer, C. R. (1994, April). *Reducing the toll: Youth suicide prevention*. Theme address presented at the 27th Annual Meeting of the American Association of Suicidology, New York.

Pfeffer, C. R., Hurt, S. W., Kakuma, T., Peskin, J. R., Siefker, C. A., & Nagabhairava, S. (1994). Suicidal children grow up: Suicidal episodes and effects of treatment during follow-up. *Journal of the American Academy of Child and Adolescent Psychiatry, 33*, 225–230.

Pfeffer, C. R., Peskin, J. R., & Siefker, C. A. (1992). Suicidal children grow up: Psychiatric treatment during follow-up period. *Journal of the American Academy of Child and Adolescent Psychiatry, 31*(4), 679–685.

Rich, A. R., Kirkpatrick-Smith, J., Bonner, R. L., & Jans, F. (1992). Gender differences in the psychosocial correlates of suicidal ideation among adolescents. *Suicide and Life-Threatening Behavior, 22*(3), 364–373.

Richman, J. (1986). *Family therapy for suicidal people*. New York: Springer Publishing.

Rotheram-Borus, M. J. (1990, October). *The treatment of adolescents who have attempted suicide*. Institute presentation at the Annual Meeting of the American Academy of Child and Adolescent Psychiatry, Chicago, IL.

Rotheram-Borus, M. J., & Trautman, P. (1988). Hopelessness, depression, and suicidal intent among adolescent suicide attempters. *Journal of the American Academy of Child and Adolescent Psychiatry, 27*, 700–704.

Rourke, B. P. (1988). Socioemotional disturbances of learning disabled children. *Journal of Consulting and Clinical Psychology, 56*(6), 801–810.

Rourke, R., Young, G., & Leenaars, A. (1989). A childhood learning disability that predisposes those afflicted to adolescent and adult depression and suicide risk. *Journal of Learning Disabilities, 22,* 169–175.

Sanborn, C. J. (1990). Gender socialization and suicide: American Association of Suicidology Presidential Address, 1989. *Suicide and Life-Threatening Behavior, 20*(2), 148–155.

Schneidman, E. S. (1985). *Definition of suicide.* New York: John Wiley & Sons.

Schneidman, E. S. (1988). Some reflections of a founder. *Suicide and Life-Threatening Behavior, 18,* 1–12.

Shaffer, D. (1974). Suicide in childhood and early adolescence. *Journal of Child Psychological Psychiatry, 15,* 275–291.

Shaffer, D. (1988). The epidemiology of teen suicide: An examination of risk factors. *Journal of Clinical Psychiatry, 49*(9, Suppl.), 36–41.

Shaffer, D., Garland, A., Gould, M., Fisher, P., & Trautman, P. (1988). Preventing teenage suicide: A critical review. *Journal of the American Academy of Child and Adolescent Psychiatry, 27*(6), 675–687.

Shafii, M., Carrigan, S., Whittinghill, J. R., & Derrick, A. (1985). Psychological autopsy of completed suicide in children and adolescents. *American Journal of Psychiatry, 142,* 1061–1064.

Simonds, J. F., McMahon, T., & Armstrong, D. (1991). Young suicide attempters compared with a control group: Psychological, affective, and attitudinal variables. *Suicide and Life-Threatening Behavior, 21*(2), 134–151.

Slater, J., & Depue, R. A. (1981). The contribution of environmental events and social support to serious suicide attempts in primary depressive disorder. *Journal of Abnormal Psychology, 90,* 275–285.

Smith, K., & Crawford, S. (1986). Suicidal behavior among normal high school students. *Suicide and Life-Threatening Behavior, 16,* 313–325.

Swedo, S. E. (1989). Postdischarge therapy of hospitalized adolescent suicide attempters. *Journal of Adolescent Health Care, 10,* 541–544.

Trautman, P. D., & Rotheram, M. J. (1986, October). Referral failure among adolescent suicide attempters. Poster presented at the Annual Meeting of the American Academy of Child Psychiatry, Los Angeles, CA.

Wade, N. L. (1987). Suicide as a resolution of separation-individuation among adolescent girls. *Adolescence, 22*(85), 169–177.

Yufit, R. I. (1991). American Association of Suicidology Presidential Address: Suicide Assessment in the 1990s. *Suicide and Life-Threatening Behavior, 21*(2), 152–163.

Zimmerman, J. K. (1991). Crossing the desert alone: An etiological model of female adolescent suicidality. In C. Gilligan, A. G. Rogers, & D. L. Tolman (Eds.), *Women, girls, and psychotherapy: Reframing resistance* (pp. 223–240). New York: Haworth Press.

Zimmerman, J. K. (1993a, April). *Loss and disconnection in adolescent suicide: A cross-cultural and female developmental perspective.* Presented as part of a panel at the 26th Annual Conference of the American Association of Suicidology, San Francisco.

Zimmerman, J. K. (1993b, April). *Adolescent suicidality and neuropsychological impairment: The development of a brief neuropsychological screening battery.* Presented at the 26th Annual Conference of the American Association of Suicidology, San Francisco.

Zimmerman, J. K. (1994, April). *The do-gooder with two faces: The case of a 17-year-old male suicide attempter.* Paper presented at the 27th Annual Meeting of the American Association of Suicidology, New York.

Zimmerman, J. K., & Morledge, J. (1992). *Prevalence of specific suicidal behaviors in a high school sample: A replication and extension.* Unpublished manuscript.

2

Suicidal Behavior in Adolescents
A Review of Risk and Protective Factors

DANIEL E. GROSZ,
JAMES K. ZIMMERMAN, AND
GREGORY M. ASNIS

The past decade has been characterized by many efforts to place adolescent suicide prevention on the public health agenda. For example, in the late 1980s, a task force on youth suicide, convened by the Department of Health and Human Services, led to a comprehensive review of risk factors and prevention strategies addressing the serious problem of suicide among young people (Alcohol, Drug Abuse, and Mental Health Administration, 1989).

Such efforts have been spurred by the fact that suicidal behavior among adolescents has become a relatively common phenomenon in the United States. Recent national surveys conducted by the Gallup Organization among randomly selected youngsters 13 to 19 years of age demonstrated that 5 to 6 percent have tried to commit suicide, 12 to 15 percent have come very close to trying to commit suicide, and approximately 60 percent personally knew a teenager who attempted suicide. In addition, over 50 percent reported intermittent suicidal ideation (Gallup, 1991, 1994), while other studies suggest that this incidence may be even higher (Harkavy Friedman, Asnis, Boeck, & DiFiore, 1987; Smith & Crawford, 1986; Zimmerman & Morledge, 1992). Completed suicide is currently the third leading cause of death among adolescents ages 15 to 19 in this country (11.3 deaths per

100,000 population), slightly behind accidents and homicide (National Center for Health Statistics, 1991).

Though completed suicide in teenagers is a relatively rare event, suicide attempts among teenagers are much more frequent. Harkavy Friedman and associates (1987) conducted a study in a large urban high school using a paper-and-pencil questionnaire about suicidal behaviors. This survey, administered anonymously, found that nearly 9 percent of adolescent respondents acknowledged a previous suicide attempt, with over half of the attempters having made multiple attempts. In the Gallup Organization's (1991, 1994) mail-in surveys, statistically similar rates of suicide attempts were found. Further, it has been estimated that for every completed suicide among adolescents, there are 50 to 200 suicide attempts (Berman & Jobes, 1991; Hawton, 1986; Orbach & Bar-Joseph, 1993; Pfeffer, 1986).

Moreover, adolescents who have already attempted suicide constitute a subgroup of teenagers at higher risk. A controlled psychological autopsy study of completed suicides in adolescence showed that 20 percent of males and 30 percent of females had made a previous suicide attempt (Shaffer, Garland, Gould, Fisher, & Trautman, 1988). Follow-up studies of adolescent suicide attempters admitted to a psychiatric hospital found an 8 to 11 percent mortality from suicide for boys and 1 percent for girls (Motto, 1984; Otto, 1972). The high risk for suicide among hospitalized adolescent suicide attempters, however, might be related to previous suicidal behavior or to severe psychopathology in general, since for nonhospitalized adolescent suicide attempters, the rates of completed suicide on follow-up were at least ten times lower (Hawton, 1987). Nevertheless, these data corroborate other studies that suggest that, as opposed to targeting services directed at a completely unselected group of teenagers, a greater preventive impact might well evolve from services directed at teenagers, particularly boys, who have made a previous suicide attempt and were hospitalized in a psychiatric facility (Pfeffer et al., 1993; Shaffer et al., 1988).

For several reasons, it may be advantageous to target for suicide prevention programs individuals who have already attempted suicide or expressed suicidal thoughts or wishes. Not only are they at higher risk for later death by suicide, but they are identified relatively easily, since many will be brought to an emergency room after their attempt or verbalization (Kennedy, Kreitman, & Ovenstone, 1974). Further, directing a preventive effort at individuals who have overtly demonstrated suicidal behavior avoids concerns that the idea of suicide is being introduced to them by the effort itself (Shaffer et al., 1988). This approach also conserves limited staff and economic resources, directing them to a subgroup that is more likely to be in need of mental health services (Shaffer et al., 1990).

Given all this, a major undertaking in recent years has been to better comprehend the underpinnings of adolescent suicide behavior. Research and clinical programs have been implemented with the intent to identify more rapidly and accurately those adolescents at risk for suicide, in order to provide them with timely and effective interventions. A number of variables have been identified as risk factors for attempted and completed suicide in adolescents.

Moreover, in considering the essential elements of effective interventions for youth suicide, it is important to identify not only risk factors—factors that have been found to correlate positively with suicidal behavior—but also protective factors—those that have been found to correlate negatively with suicidal behavior. Successful treatment strategies developed for suicidal teenagers can be conceptualized as interventions that decrease the impact of risk factors and enhance the role of protective factors.

The following section reviews the salient issues raised by studies focused on risk factors. Subsequent sections consider factors that may attenuate adolescent suicidality and present models that have attempted to integrate risk and protective factors.

RISK FACTORS

It is widely accepted that suicidal behavior in youth has multiple biopsychosocial risk factors. (For more extensive reviews, see Berman & Jobes, 1991; Davidson & Gould, 1989; Pfeffer et al., 1991; Pfeffer et al., 1993.) It is important to note, however, that it is as yet unclear whether suicide attempts and completed suicide can be conceptualized as distinct behaviors (Carlson & Cantwell, 1982) or as occurring in a continuum (Pfeffer, 1986) with common antecedents (Felner, Adan, & Silverman, 1992). Some studies (Brent & Kolko, 1990; Brent et al., 1986) comparing adolescent suicide attempters to suicide victims and controls support the notion that these are distinct but overlapping populations; among the attempters, those who made more lethal attempts were most like the suicide completers. It is therefore difficult to discern and delineate risk factors for completed suicide per se from those producing emotional turmoil, mental disturbance, and suicidal behavior in general.

The following consideration of risk for suicide in adolescence thus focuses on those factors that appear to predict or correlate with suicidality overall, with particular attention to findings related to suicide attempters, since that is the central interest of this volume.

Demographic Risk Factors

Age, Gender, and Race

The peak age for suicide attempts both in females and males is the period between ages 15 and 24 (Schuckit & Schuckit, 1989), although for suicide completers this peak occurs in the elderly (National Center for Health Statistics, 1992). Male suicides in the 15- to 19-year-old age group outnumber females by approximately four to one (Berman & Jobes, 1991; Rosenberg, Smith, Davidson, & Conn, 1987). Adolescent suicide attempters are more likely to be females, and their preferred method tends to be drug overdoses. Conversely, the paradigmatic adolescent suicide completer is a white male employing a more lethal method (such as firearms or hanging).

White male adolescents consistently have the highest rate of suicide among male and female whites and blacks, with black males having the second highest rate and black females having the lowest (Garrison, 1992; Holinger, 1989); thus, there is an apparent race-gender interaction between these subgroups. Further, rates among Hispanics generally have been found to be lower than those for whites (Smith, Mercy, & Rosenberg, 1986; Sorenson & Golding, 1988), although one study found parity in rates between Mexican-American and white adolescent males (Smith et al., 1986). However, few studies have separated Hispanics by cultural subgroup, nation of origin, or immigrant status; one that endeavored to do this reported few clear differences between whites, blacks, and various Hispanic subgroups (Vega, Gil, Warheit, Apospori, & Zimmerman, 1993).

Secular Trends

Between the 1950s and the 1980s, the rate of completed adolescent suicide tripled, largely due to an increase in suicides among white males (Garrison, 1992); since the early 1980s, this rate has stabilized at approximately 13 completed suicides per 100,000 population (Holinger, 1989). Possible explanations for this trebling have included cohort effects (Holinger, 1989; Murphy & Wetzel, 1980; Solomon & Hellon, 1980), unemployment rates (Stack, 1993), and a lack of access to external sources of self-esteem in the context of increased competition for finite resources in times of increasing population. (See Garrison, 1992, for a more complete review of these issues.)

There has been an increase in other suicidal behaviors in comparison with other age groups as well (National Center for Health Statistics, 1991). This upsurge has been linked to parallel increases in the rates of depression and substance abuse in youth born after World War II (Brent & Kolko, 1990). These trends suggest either a possible causal link among depression, substance abuse, and suicidality, or a multicollinear relationship among the three. One hypothesis suggests an involvement of the serotonergic neurochemical system (Lester, 1988; see also the section "Biological Risk Factors" later).

Psychosocial Risk Factors

Family Risk Factors

Several categories of family factors have been associated with suicidal behavior among youth. First, there are stresses involving changes in the composition of the family subsequent to deaths, parental separation or divorce, and other losses. Adolescents who have undergone these adjustments in their family life have been shown repeatedly to be more at risk for suicidal behavior (Cohen-Sandler, Berman, & King, 1982; Garfinkel, Froese, & Hood, 1982; Isherwood, Adam, & Hornblow, 1982; Stanley & Barter, 1970).

Second, family violence involving physical and sexual abuse has been related to adolescent suicidality (Shafii, Carrigan, Whittinghill, & Derrick, 1985; Deykin, Alpert, & McNamara, 1985). Deykin and colleagues found, in a sample of 159 adolescents seen in a hospital emergency room subsequent to a suicide attempt, that approximately one in eight of these attempts could be attributed etiologically to parental abuse. Moreover, these suicide attempters were three to six times more likely to have come to the attention of social service agencies in the past as a result of suspected parental abuse or neglect than were nonsuicidal controls who were also seen in the same emergency room. Perhaps collinear with physical and sexual abuse is the finding that family discord and low cohesiveness also are associated with suicidal behavior in adolescents (Asarnow, Carlson, & Guthrie, 1987; Fremouw, Callahan, & Kashden, 1993; Jaffe, Offord, & Boyle, 1988; King, Raskin, Gdowski, Butkus, & Opipari, 1990; Rich, Fowler, Fogarty, & Young, 1988; Rubenstein, Heeren, Housman, Rubin, & Stechler, 1989).

Third, symptoms of depression, suicidal behavior, or other psychiatric illness have been found to be more common in the families of suicidal children and adolescents (Brent, Kolko, Allan, & Brown, 1990; Garfinkel et al., 1982; Pfeffer, 1989a; Shafii et al., 1985; Shaffer, 1974, 1988).

Stressful Life Events

A number of studies, both of adolescent suicide attempters alone and in comparison with control groups, suggest high rates of recent life stress and of early family disruptions among adolescent suicide attempters (Paykel, 1989). For example, suicide attempters have had more stressful life events in the 12 months prior to hospitalization than did psychiatric controls (Brent & Kolko, 1990; Cohen-Sandler et al., 1982) and more major life events in general from early to middle adolescence than normal controls (Jacobs, 1971; Pfeffer, 1989a, 1989b). Negative life stress has been shown to predict suicidal ideation in college students (Rich & Bonner, 1987), and total life stress has correlated with suicidal behavior among high school students (Rubenstein et al., 1989).

Particular stressors implicated include conflict with parents, loss of a boyfriend or girlfriend, school changes, and loss of a parent due to divorce or death (Garfinkel et al., 1982; Hawton, O'Grady, Osborne, & Cole, 1982; Kosky, 1983; Pfeffer, 1989a; Pfeffer, Newcorn, Kaplan, Mizruchi, & Plutchik, 1988). However, as these stresses also are generic to adolescence, affecting countless teenagers every day who *do not* respond with suicidal behavior, it is essential to look beyond the stressor per se to some feature of the individual's personality or to a coexisting mental illness (Shaffer et al., 1988). This issue is considered more fully in the section entitled "The Interrelationship of Risk and Protective Factors."

Exposure to Physical or Sexual Abuse

Unfortunately, abuse is an all-too-frequent occurrence in childhood and adolescence. It has been estimated recently that 34 percent of adolescents in outpatient treatment have experienced physical abuse and 44 percent have suffered sexual abuse (Lipschitz, Kaplan, & Asnis, 1994). Battered children have been reported to have a significantly higher incidence of suicide attempts and other self-destructive behaviors (41 percent) than comparison groups of neglected children (17 percent) and normal controls (7 percent) (Green, 1978). A number of other studies have found a significant association of suicide attempts and abuse in adolescents (Deykin et al., 1985; Rich et al., 1988; Sansonnet-Hayden, Haley, & Marriage, 1987).

Imitation and Contagion

Several lines of evidence support the contention that imitation can play a role in the pathogenesis of adolescent suicidal behavior (Davidson & Gould, 1989; Gould & Shaffer, 1986; Gould, Wallenstein, & Kleinman, 1990; Phillips, Lesyna, & Paight, 1992; Stack, Gundlach, & Reeves, 1994). Exposure to suicide usually has been divided into direct person-to-person exposure (referring to the presence of suicidal behavior within the family or other individuals close to the identified patient) and indirect exposure (referring to influence through the media). Media exposure includes the coverage of fictional and nonfictional suicides (Davidson & Gould, 1989).

Most evidence for an imitation hypothesis comes from epidemiological studies of suicide rates before and after indirect exposure due to coverage of selected suicides at the local and national level (Gould & Shaffer, 1986). There is an apparent relationship between an increase in suicides and the publicity given in the media to suicides of well-known celebrities, particularly those in politics and entertainment (Stack, 1987, 1993). There is also some evidence that an upsurge in suicides does not occur if suicides are not given major (front-page) attention in the media (Phillips et al., 1992).

Some studies have found an increase in suicides following televised fictional accounts of suicide, although there are mitigating factors such as the way in which a suicide is presented and what information accompanies the broadcast (Gould & Shaffer, 1986; Gould, Shaffer, & Kleinman, 1988; Häfner & Schmidke, 1989; Phillips & Paight, 1987; Schmidke & Häfner, 1988). Recent research also has suggested a relationship between the "heavy metal" music subculture and suicidality in adolescents (Stack, Gundlach, & Reeves, 1994).

Regarding direct exposure, there is evidence that suicidal behavior in the family increases the risk of adolescent suicide (Pfeffer, 1989a, 1989b), as does exposure to suicidal behavior in peers (Lewinsohn, 1994).

Some concern has been expressed as a result of studies that suggested suicide prevention programs for adolescents in schools are ineffective or even negative and may actually *increase* suicidality among those at high risk (Shaffer et al., 1988; Shaffer, Garland, & Bacon, 1989; Shaffer et al., 1990). However, other studies have found positive effects of suicide awareness and prevention programs in schools (Abbey, Madsen, & Polland, 1989; Nelson, 1987; Spirito, Overholser, Ashworth, Morgan, & Benedict-Drew, 1988). Thus, it is unclear whether there is an imitation or contagion effect in this regard, and further research appears necessary to clarify the issue.

Social Skills, Problem Solving, and Support

Social Skills

Some studies have suggested that impaired social skills and poor peer relationships are associated with suicide attempts in adolescence (Asarnow et al., 1987; Barter, Swaback, & Todd, 1968; Crumley, 1979; Pfeffer et al., 1993; Tischler, McKenry, & Morgan, 1981), although such findings are controversial. Adolescent suicide attempters manifested more frequent and more serious peer problems than either nonsuicidal psychiatric patients or nonhospitalized controls (Topol & Reznikoff, 1982). Further, recidivists following discharge from psychiatric treatment reported significantly fewer peer interactions than first-time attempters (Stanley & Barter, 1970), and a strong relationship has been found between chronically impaired social adjustment, mood disorders, and suicide (Puig-Antich et al., 1985a, 1985b). However, other studies using global measures of social adaptation found no association between social impairment and suicidality (Brent, Zelenak, Bukstein, & Brown, 1990b; Cohen-Sandler et al., 1982; Kosky, Silburn, & Zubrick, 1986). More precise measures of social adjustment may be required to parse out the specific attributes of social environments, and ensuing social difficulties, which cause the eruption of suicidal behavior in adolescents.

Problem-Solving Skills

Clum and colleagues have suggested an interactional model of suicidality, maintaining that suicide risk increases when negative life stresses mount in an individual with poor problem-solving skills and deficient coping abilities, leading to depression, hopelessness, and suicidal behavior (Clum, Patsiokas, & Luscomb, 1979; Schotte & Clum, 1982; Yang & Clum, 1994). Studies have found that such a model applies to college students (Rich & Bonner, 1987; Schotte & Clum, 1982) and in some components to hospitalized suicidal adolescents (Fremouw et al., 1993). Thus, adequate and effective problem-solving abilities may also attenuate the impact of otherwise suicidogenic agents.

Social Support

A lack of social support has been suggested as a risk factor for suicide in adolescents (Bonner & Rich, 1988; King et al., 1990; Lewinsohn, 1994; Pfeffer et al., 1993; Rich & Bonner, 1987; Rudd, 1990; Yang & Clum, 1994); conversely, adequate social support has been suggested as protective against suicide (Pfeffer et al., 1993). Rudd (1990) proposed that social support may be a moderator between life stress and suicidality, such that higher and more stable levels of support may mitigate the impact of life stresses.

Psychiatric Risk Factors

Mood Disorders

There is clearly a strong association between mood disorders and suicidality. Mood disorders consistently have been found to be associated with suicidal ideation, suicide attempts, and completed suicide in adolescents (Brent et al., 1988; Carlson & Cantwell, 1982; Lewinsohn, 1994; Otto, 1972; Pfeffer et al., 1988; Pfeffer et al., 1993; Robbins & Alessi, 1985; Shafii et al., 1985; Swanson, Linskey, Quintero-Salinas, Pumariega, & Holzer, 1992; Welner, Welner, & Fishman, 1979). Depressive disorders are also overrepresented among suicide attempters admitted to a psychiatric facility (Friedman, Arnoff, & Clarkin, 1983; Robbins & Alessi, 1985). However, since the majority of depressed youth never attempt or complete suicide (Brent & Kolko, 1990), it is clear that other factors must come into play in the causality of suicidal behavior in depressed adolescents. These include other risk factors

discussed in this chapter (e.g., hopelessness, impaired social adjustment, poor problem-solving skills, and genetic and biological factors),
plus protective factors that may prove suicidolytic in some individuals.

Previous Suicidality

A past history of suicidality has been shown in a number of studies
to be a strong predictor of future suicidality in adolescents (Cohen-
Sandler et al., 1982; Garrison, Addy, Jackson, McKeown, & Waller,
1991; Pfeffer et al., 1993). Clearly, suicidal behavior increases the risk
of eventual death by suicide, particularly among those individuals who
have been psychiatrically hospitalized (Kuperman, Black, & Burnst,
1988; Pfeffer et al., 1993).

Hopelessness

Although many studies in the adult population have indicated that the
factor of hopelessness is a more decisive predictor of suicidality than
is depression in general (Beck, 1986; Beck, Steer, Beck, & Newman,
1993; Fawcett et al., 1990; Wetzel, Margulies, Davis, & Karam, 1980),
this finding is more equivocal in adolescents. Asarnow and Guthrie
(1989) found a positive relationship between suicidal ideation and
hopelessness in child psychiatric inpatients, as did Fremouw, Callahan, and Kashden (1993), comparing hospitalized adolescents with
normal controls. Yang and Clum (1994) likewise found such a relationship in Asian students in the United States. However, such an association was not found in normal children (Cole, 1989; Pfeffer et al., 1988)
or in urban female suicidal adolescents (Rotheram-Borus, Trautman,
Dopkins, & Shrout, 1990). Rather than appearing as a general risk
factor, as it seems to be with adults, the association among depression,
hopelessness, and suicidality in adolescents may vary according
to specific characteristics of subject samples (Cole, 1988; Holden,
Mendonca, & Serin, 1989).

Conduct and Personality Disorders

Clinical experience suggests that personality traits already may be
identified by adolescence. However, since personality is still in the
process of development in teenagers, it is unclear whether personality
disorders can be diagnosed reliably before adulthood. Despite this
limitation, some investigators have begun using semistructured interviews with adolescents to study the role of DSM Axis II pathology

(American Psychiatric Association, 1987, 1994) in adolescent suicide attempters (Brent et al., 1990; Johnson & Brent, 1991).

Among adults, it is well documented that certain personality disorders, in particular antisocial and borderline, constitute a risk factor for suicidal behavior (Frances & Blumenthal, 1989). In a sample of adult psychiatric outpatients, it was demonstrated that almost all suicide attempters had a comorbid Axis II diagnosis, regardless of their diagnosis on Axis I, suggesting a key role for personality disorders in suicidal behaviors (Sanderson, Friedman, Wetzler, Kaplan, & Asnis, 1992).

Though conduct disorder is not considered a personality disorder, it has been shown that a diagnosis of conduct disorder before age 15 is the best predictor for the development of antisocial personality (Robins, 1978). Psychological autopsy studies show that a diagnosis of conduct disorder is one of the main risk factors for completed suicide, in particular among males (Shaffer et al., 1988). In addition, conduct-disordered adolescent inpatients are significantly more suicidal than patients with major depression, even though they are significantly less depressed (Apter, Bleich, Plutchik, Mendelsohn, & Tyano, 1988).

Substance Abuse

Many studies have found higher rates of suicide among alcoholics and substance abusers (Lester, 1992). Suicidal ideation and attempts are associated with both alcohol and substance abuse in adolescents (Farberow, Litman, & Nelson, 1988; Kirkpatrick-Smith, Rich, Bonner, & Jans, 1989; Vega et al., 1993), with intoxication with alcohol or drugs often immediately preceding suicidal behavior. In some instances, this relates to suicide attempts among alcohol or drug abusers, but in others it reflects the use of substances as part of the attempt itself (Schuckit & Schuckit, 1989). Garfinkel, Froese, and Hood (1982) found a tenfold higher rate of recent alcohol or drug use in adolescent suicide attempters than in controls. Substance abuse in depressed adolescents appears both to increase the risk for multiple attempts and to add to the seriousness of the attempt (Robbins & Alessi, 1985).

Genetic Risk Factors

Several lines of evidence tend to support the role of genetic risk factors for suicidal behavior. Twin studies show higher concordance for suicidal behavior in monozygotic versus dizygotic twins (Roy, 1992). Adoption studies found that there were significantly higher suicide rates in the biological relatives of adoptees who had completed suicide, as compared to matched adopted controls (Kety, 1986; Schulsinger, Kety, Rosenthal, & Wender, 1979). This finding was true for biological families of adoptees with or without a history of a psychiatric illness, suggesting that the risk for suicide was at least partly genetic (Mann, DeMeo, Keilp, & McBride, 1989). One hypothesis is that this risk may relate to an inability to control impulsive behavior (Kety, 1986).

Among the Amish, a group characterized by very strong family ties and religious beliefs that vehemently condemn suicide, it was found that all the 26 suicides during the last century had been among members of only four families (Egeland & Sussex, 1985). Though these families had high rates of mood disorders, there were other families with high prevalence of mood disorders but with no history of suicide. This finding suggests that there may be a separate pattern of inheritance for suicide.

In studies of youth, family history data have shown that completed and attempted suicide is significantly higher among the first-degree relatives of adolescent suicide victims (Roy, 1992; Shaffer, 1974; Shaffer et al., 1988; Shafii et al., 1985), adolescent suicide attempters seen in clinical settings (Garfinkel et al., 1982; Tischler, McKenry, & Morgan, 1981), and adolescent suicide attempters from a randomly selected high school sample (Harkavy Friedman et al., 1987).

Biological Risk Factors

Recent attention has been given to biological factors as constituting another risk factor for suicidal behavior. Most of the research in this regard has been done with adults. A number of biological hypotheses have been proposed to explain the neurobiological basis for suicidal behaviors, the most widely accepted of which has been the serotonin hypothesis, although recent evidence also has suggested a relationship with diminished central dopamine neurotransmission in suicidal depressed patients (Roy, 1994).

The serotonin hypothesis suggests that suicidal behavior is associated with a serotonin deficit or a decrease in serotonin functioning. Findings supporting this hypothesis include: the presence of low concentrations of the serotonin (5-HT) metabolite, 5-hydroxyindolacetic acid (5-HIAA), in the cerebrospinal fluid (CSF) of suicide attempters and victims regardless of their psychiatric diagnosis (Åsberg, 1991;

Åsberg, Träskman, & Thoren, 1976; van Praag et al., 1990); a decrease in presynaptic imipramine binding, a platelet marker believed to reflect central serotonin functioning; an increase of 5-HT_2 receptors in platelets of suicidal patients (McBride, Brown, & DeMeo, 1987); and an increase in the density of postsynaptic 5-HT_2 receptor binding in brains of suicide victims (Stanley, 1989), believed to be compensatory, secondary to a 5-HT_2 presynaptic deficit. Recently, low CSF 5-HIAA has been found to predict suicide risk in the short term among mood disordered psychiatric inpatients (Nordström et al., 1994).

Further evidence of altered 5-HT_2 metabolism in suicide attempters comes from studies using neuroendocrine challenges such as L-tryptophan, a serotonin precursor, and fenfluramine, a serotonin releaser and agonist (Meltzer & Lowy, 1989).

Inspired by findings in adult subjects, a small number of preliminary investigations of biological markers in suicidal adolescents have been undertaken. Ryan and associates (1988) reported that adolescents with major depressive disorder (MDD) and a history of suicide attempts had a blunted growth hormone (GH) secretion after a desipramine (DMI) challenge, as compared to MDD nonsuicidal patients and normal adolescent controls. The GH response to DMI is predominantly under 5-HT regulation. Thus, this finding supports a 5-HT dysfunction for adolescent suicide attempters.

Disturbances in 5-HT metabolism also have been studied more directly in adolescent suicide attempters. Biegon, Grinspoon, and Blumenfeld (1990) measured platelet 5-HT_2 receptor binding in a group of 22 young suicidal subjects and 19 normal controls. Platelet 5-HT_2 receptor binding in the suicidal subjects was significantly higher than in controls. A preliminary report by Greenhill and associates (1991) reported that nine inpatient suicidal subjects with MDD had relatively low CSF 5-HIAA values; CSF 5-HIAA changes after treatment with fluoxetine correlated negatively with the prolactin response to fenfluramine among the same subjects. Thus, patients with a very low prolactin response to fenfluramine—representing a subgroup with decreased 5-HT functioning—did best with a serotonin-specific antidepressant treatment, fluoxetine. The latter suggests that a subgroup of suicidal adolescents can be identified with a biological laboratory test and therefore potentially can receive selective medications for their pathological behaviors.

PROTECTIVE FACTORS IN
ADOLESCENT SUICIDE

To this point, this chapter has focused predominantly on risk factors for adolescent suicidal behaviors. Within the last ten years there also has been a burgeoning interest in identifying factors that militate against adolescent suicidal behaviors (Rolf, Masten, Cichetti, Neuchterlein, & Weintraub, 1990). These latter protective factors include variables such as the presence of social support and individual adaptive skills (Pfeffer, 1989a, 1989b; Pfeffer et al., 1993) and are essential to an understanding of why some children adapt in positive ways even within stressful environments while others develop behavioral disorders. Research in this realm also contributes to the differentiation between vulnerable and stress-resistant individuals, their environments, and the interactions that predict successful and unsuccessful adaptation. Thus, information on risk and protective factors together also may be instrumental in the development of prevention strategies for persons at risk (Institute of Medicine, 1989).

THE INTERRELATIONSHIP OF RISK
AND PROTECTIVE FACTORS

Models explaining the interaction of risk and protective factors for youth suicide have been proposed. Shaffer and colleagues (1988) assume that suicide does not occur randomly but only strikes certain individuals who are predisposed, and that these individuals will commit suicide only if there are co-occurring triggering stresses and method opportunities. The individual predispositions include a major depressive disorder and certain personality types, and a suicide often will take place shortly after a stressful event induces some extreme emotion, most commonly fear or rage. Distorted affect also may follow from a depressed mood or intoxication with drugs or alcohol. Finally, the means of committing suicide must be at hand. This model assumes that very few individuals other than those just delineated will be at risk for completed suicide.

Clum and colleagues (Clum et al., 1979; Schotte & Clum, 1982; Yang & Clum, 1994) proposed a diathesis-stress model of the etiology of suicide, such that suicidal behavior would be the consequence of increased stress in individuals who had poor inter-personal problem-solving skills. Another diathesis-stress model, de-lineated by Rudd (1990), suggested a similar relationship among inadequate social supports, life stress, and suicide.

A two-stage model of suicide and violence (Plutchik & van Praag, 1986; Plutchik, van Praag, & Conte, 1989) also has been applied to explain adolescent suicidal behavior (Apter et al., 1988; Grosz, Blackwood, Finkelstein, & Plutchik, 1991). This model is based on the concept that both suicidal and violent behaviors are built on a foundation of underlying aggressive impulses. A small number of triggers—such as, threat, challenge, insult, loss of control, and a de-crease in one's hierarchical position—may generate such impulses. The aggression thus generated is attenuated or amplified by other variables. Attenuators include timidity, isolation, being appeased by others, close family ties, having sex, and being distracted. Amplifiers include school problems, distrust, access to weapons, and probably substance abuse. Yet another set of opposing variables determines the direction of the aggression (inward or outward). Factors tending to direct violence inward are depression, a large number of life prob-lems, hopelessness, and recent psychiatric symptoms. Those direct-ing the aggressive impulse outward include the trait of impulsivity, legal trouble, menstrual problems, and recent life stress (Plutchik & van Praag, 1986). Since overt suicidal behavior may modify the orig-inal triggers of the suicidal behavior by communicating within the social network, a "behavioral homeostatic feedback system" may en-sue (Apter et al., 1988).

A similar model of opposing vectors indicating risk and protective factors for the expression of youth suicidal behavior was suggested by Pfeffer (1989a, 1989b). For example, qualities of a supportive individ-ual such as an ability to provide empathy, consistent availability, ca-pacity to set limits and offer structure, and ability to gratify individual needs to enhance self-esteem may be important social support vectors that might attenuate suicidal behavior. Factors such as family disorga-nization, parental psychopathology, and family violence are vectors that would enhance suicidal behavior.

Another model (Blumenthal, 1990; Blumenthal & Kupfer, 1988) delineated five domains organized as a matrix or multiaxial set to en-compass most of the risk factors for suicidal behavior. These domains include psychiatric diagnosis, personality traits, psychosocial factors, life events and chronic medical illness, and biological, family history, and genetic factors.

Whether a model of risk should be a series of interlocking Venn diagrams, a diathesis-stress model, or an additive one, it does appear that a central clinical research strategy will be to develop weights for each of its major components. For example, in applying a model, the breakup of a relationship might be a final humiliating experience that triggers a depressive episode in a young person with a family history of mood disorder. Such an individual also may have poor social supports, which interact with the other identified risk factors to increase the individual's vulnerability to suicide.

Perhaps the salient question is this: At what level and in what degree do each of these factors contribute to suicide potential? Or is the degree of overlap of all factors the most important criterion? Alternatively, we may wish to pose such a question as: What makes 15 percent of the people who suffer from a mood disorder end their lives by suicide while the other 85 percent do not? Using this overlapping model, we may learn that the subgroup of mood-disordered patients who commit suicide has a greater interdigitation of other risk domains, such as increased hopelessness, impulsiveness, decreased social supports, recent humiliating life experiences, and/or a greater likelihood of a family history of mood disorder or suicidal behavior.

There is no doubt that adolescent suicidal behavior is a multidetermined phenomenon. However, despite the proliferation of various models, the studies just reviewed generally do not address hypotheses about the mechanisms underlying the interaction of risk and protective factors. It still remains unclear how multiple risk and protective factors interact. Since both risk and protective factors coexist at any one time, the strength of the suicidal impulse could be a vectorial sum of these opposing forces. For example, early loss of social supports may be an important stress that affects the development of personality characteristics and/or biological systems and thereby enhances chronic vulnerability to suicidal behavior. On the other hand, an acute loss of social supports may alter existing psychological and/or biological functioning. This may create a temporary acute crisis in ego functioning that affects the quality of a youngster's affect regulation, impulse control, judgment, cognition, and fantasies (Pfeffer, 1989b).

CONCLUSION

The foregoing is testament to how much has been learned in recent years about what factors increase the likelihood of suicidal behavior in adolescents and what factors decrease that likelihood. Moreover, some depth of understanding has been developed regarding the interplay between risk and protective factors. The promise in this endeavor is that prevention and intervention services will become more finely honed and precise, leading to a clear decrease in the incidence of suicide in the young.

Nevertheless, much work is still to be done, as indicated by the fact that the rate of suicide in adolescents, although slightly lower than it was in the late 1970s, has stabilized but not decreased in recent years. It is also unclear whether this stabilization of rates is in fact due to public awareness and prevention and intervention programs, or whether it is a consequence of other anomalous factors, such as population demographics. The true test of the understanding of risk and protective factors and their relationship to prevention of adolescent suicide will come in the further definition and refinement of theoretical models, based on empirical findings, and in the successful application of these models in clinical practice. Only then, when comprehension of the issues is clarified and the successful interventions are the proof of that understanding, will it be possible to know definitively that progress has been made. For the interim, then, work must continue and expand in refining theoretical models, designing and implementing programs that derive from these models, and evaluating the outcome of these interventions. The inspiration for this work will be the knowledge that there are lives to save, tragedies to avert, and futures to enhance.

REFERENCES

Abbey, K. J., Madsen, C. H., & Polland, R. (1989). Short-term suicide awareness curriculum. *Suicide and Life-Threatening Behavior, 19,* 216–222.

Alcohol, Drug Abuse, and Mental Health Administration. (1989). *Report of the Secretary's Task Force on Youth Suicide (vol. I): Overview and recommendations.* DHHS Pub. No. (ADM)89-1621. Washington, DC: U.S. Government Printing Office.

American Psychiatric Association. (1987). *Diagnostic and statistical manual of mental disorders* (3rd ed. rev.) (DSM-IIIR). Washington, DC: American Psychiatric Association.

American Psychiatric Association. (1994). *Diagnostic and statistical manual of mental disorders* (4th ed.) (DSM-IV). Washington, DC: American Psychiatric Association.

Apter, A., Bleich, A., Plutchik, R., Mendelsohn, S., & Tyano, S. (1988). Suicidal behavior, depression, and conduct disorder in hospitalized adolescents. *Journal of the American Academy of Child and Adolescent Psychiatry, 27*(6), 696–699.

Asarnow, J. R., Carlson, G. A., & Guthrie, D. (1987). Coping strategies, self-perception, hopelessness, and perceived family environments in depressed and suicidal children. *Journal of Consulting and Clinical Psychology, 55,* 361–366.

Asarnow, J. R., & Guthrie, D. (1989). Suicidal behavior, depression, and hopelessness in child psychiatric inpatients: A replication and extension. *Journal of Clinical Child Psychology, 18,* 129–136.

Åsberg, M. L. (1991). Neurotransmitter monoamine metabolites in the cerebrospinal fluid as risk factors for suicidal behavior. In L. Davidson & M. Linnoila (Eds.), (1989). *Report of the Secretary's Task Force on Youth Suicide: (Vol. 2). Risk factors for youth suicide* (pp. 193–212). DHHS Pub. No. (ADM)89-1622. Washington, DC: U.S. Government Printing Office.

Åsberg, M. L., Träskman, L., & Thoren, P. (1976). 5-H1AA in the cerebrospinal fluid: A biochemical suicide predictor? *Archives of General Psychiatry, 33,* 1193–1197.

Barter, J. T., Swaback, D. O., & Todd, D. (1968). Adolescent suicide attempts: A follow-up study of hospitalized patients. *Archives of General Psychiatry, 19,* 523–527.

Beck, A. T. (1986). Hopelessness as a predictor of eventual suicide. In J. J. Mann & M. Stanley (Eds.), *Psychobiology of suicidal behavior* (pp. 90–96). New York: Academy of Sciences.

Beck, A. T., Steer, R. A., Beck, J. S., & Newman, C. F. (1993). Hopelessness, depression, suicidal ideation, and clinical diagnosis of depression. *Suicide and Life-Threatening Behavior, 23*(2), 139–145.

Berman, A. L., & Jobes, D. A. (1991). *Adolescent suicide: Assessment and intervention.* Washington, DC: American Psychological Association.

Biegon, A., Grinspoon, A., & Blumenfeld, B. (1990). Increased serotonin-2 receptor binding on blood platelets of suicidal men. *Psychopharmacology, 100,* 165–167.

Blumenthal, S. J. (1990). Youth suicide: The physician's role in suicide prevention. *Journal of the American Medical Association, 264,* 3194–3196.

Blumenthal, S. J., & Kupfer, D. J. (1988). Overview of early detection and treatment strategies for suicidal behavior in young people. *Journal of Youth and Adolescence, 17*(1), 1–23.

Bonner, R. L., & Rich, A. R. (1988). Negative life stress, social problem-solving self-appraisal, and hopelessness: Implications for suicide research. *Cognitive Therapy and Research, 12,* 549–556.

Brent, D. A., Kalas, R., Edelbrock, C., Costello, A., Dulcan, M., & Conover, N. (1986). Psychopathology and its relationship to suicidal ideation in childhood and adolescents. *Journal of the American Academy of Child Psychiatry, 25,* 666–673.

Brent, D. A., & Kolko, D. J. (1990). Suicide and suicidal behavior in children and adolescents. In B. D. Garfinkel, G. A. Carlson, & E. B. Weller (Eds.), *Psychiatric disorders in children and adolescents.* Philadelphia, PA: W. B. Saunders.

Brent, D., Kolko, D. J., Allan, M. J., & Brown, R. V. (1990). Suicidality in affectively disordered adolescent inpatients. *Journal of the American Academy of Child and Adolescent Psychiatry, 29,* 586–593.

Brent, D. A., Perper, J. A., Goldstein, C. E., Kolko, D. J., Allan, M. J., Allman, C. J., & Zelenak, J. P. (1988). Risk factors for adolescent suicide: A comparison of adolescent suicide victims with suicidal inpatients. *Archives of General Psychiatry, 45,* 581–588.

Brent, D., Zelenak, J. P., Bukstein, O., & Brown, R. V. (1990). Reliability and validity of the structured interview for personality disorders in adolescents. *Journal of the American Academy of Child and Adolescent Psychiatry, 29*(3), 349–354.

Carlson, G. A., & Cantwell, D. P. (1982). Suicidal behavior and depression in children and adolescents. *Journal of the American Academy of Child Psychiatry, 21,* 361–368.

Clum, G., Patsiokas, A., & Luscomb, R. (1979). Empirically based comprehensive treatment program for parasuicide. *Journal of Consulting and Clinical Psychology, 47,* 937–945.

Cohen-Sandler, R., Berman, A. L., & King, R. A. (1982). Life stress and symptomatology: Determinants of suicidal behavior in children. *Journal of the American Academy of Child Psychiatry, 21,* 178–186.

Cole, D. A. (1988). Hopelessness, social desirability, depression, and parasuicide in two college student samples. *Journal of Consulting and Clinical Psychology, 56,* 131–136.

Cole, D. A. (1989). Psychopathology of adolescent suicide: Hopelessness, coping beliefs, and depression. *Journal of Abnormal Psychology, 98,* 248–255.

Crumley, F. E. (1979). Adolescent suicide attempts. *Journal of the American Medical Association, 241*(22), 2404–2407.

Davidson, L., & Gould M. (1989). Contagion as a risk factor for youth suicide. In L. Davidson & M. Linnoila (Eds.), *Report of the Secretary's Task Force on Youth Suicide: (Vol. 2). Risk factors for youth suicide* (pp. 88–109). DHHS Pub. No. (ADM)89-1622. Washington, DC: U.S. Government Printing Office.

Deykin, E. Y., Alpert, J. J., & McNamara, J. J. (1985). A pilot study of the effect of exposure to child abuse or neglect on adolescent suicidal behavior. *American Journal of Psychiatry, 142,* 1299–1303.

Egeland, J. A., & Sussex, J. N. (1985). Suicide and family loading for affective disorders. *Journal of the American Medical Association, 254,* 915–918.

Farberow, N. L., Litman, R. E., & Nelson, F. L. (1988). A survey of youth suicide in California. In R. Yufit (Ed.), *Proceedings of the 21st Annual Meeting of the American Association of Suicidology* (pp. 298–300). Denver, CO: American Association of Suicidology.

Fawcett, J., Scheftner, W. A., Fogg, L., Clark, D. C., Young, M. A., Hedeker, D., & Gibbons, R. (1990). Time-related prediction of suicide in major affective disorder. *American Journal of Psychiatry, 147,* 1189–1194.

Felner, R. D., Adan, A. M., & Silverman, M. M. (1992). Risk assessment and prevention of youth suicide in schools and educational contexts. In R. W. Maris, A. L. Berman, J. T. Maltsberger, & R. I. Yufit (Eds.), *Assessment and prediction of suicide* (pp. 420–447). New York: The Guilford Press.

Frances, A., & Blumenthal, S. J. (1989). Personality as a predictor of youthful suicide. In L. Davidson & M. Linnoila (Eds.), *Report of the Secretary's Task Force on Youth Suicide: (Vol. 2). Risk factors for youth suicide* (pp. 160–171). DHHS Pub. No. (ADM)89-1622. Washington, DC: U.S. Government Printing Office.

Fremouw, W., Callahan, T., & Kashden, J. (1993). Adolescent suicidal risk: Psychological, problem solving, and environmental factors. *Suicide and Life-Threatening Behavior, 23*(1), 46–54.

Friedman, R. C., Arnoff, M. S., & Clarkin, J. F. (1983). History of suicidal behavior in depressed borderline adolescent inpatients. *American Journal of Psychiatry, 35,* 837–844.

Gallup Organization. (1991, March). *Teenage suicide study: Executive summary.* Princeton, NJ: Gallup Organization.

Gallup Organization. (1994, June). *Teenage suicide study: Executive summary.* Princeton, NJ: Gallup Organization.

Garfinkel, B. D., Froese, A., & Hood, J. (1982). Suicide attempts in children and adolescents. *American Journal of Psychiatry, 139,* 1257–1261.

Garrison, C. Z. (1992). Demographic predictors of suicide. In R. W. Maris, A. L. Berman, J. T. Maltsberger, & R. I. Yufit (Eds.), *Assessment and prediction of suicide* (pp. 484–496). New York: The Guilford Press.

Garrison, C. Z., Addy, C. L., Jackson, K. L., McKeown, R. E., & Waller, J. L. (1991). A longitudinal study of suicidal ideation in young adolescents.

Journal of the American Academy of Child and Adolescent Psychiatry, 30, 597–603.

Gould, M., & Shaffer, D. (1986). The impact of suicide in television movies: Evidence of imitation. *New England Journal of Medicine, 315,* 690–694.

Gould, M. S., Shaffer, D., & Kleinman, M. (1988). The impact of suicide in television movies: Replication and commentary. *Suicide and Life-Threatening Behavior, 18,* 90–99.

Gould, M. S., Wallenstein, S., & Kleinman, M. (1990). Time-space clustering of teenage suicide. *American Journal of Epidemiology, 131,* 71–78.

Green, A. H. (1978). Self-destructive behavior in battered children. *American Journal of Psychiatry, 135,* 579–582.

Greenhill, L., Stanley, M., Cooper, T., Setterberg, S., Elzohairy, B., Clarvit, S., Parides, M., Shapiro, B., Cohen, L., & Shaffer, D. (1991, October). *Biological studies in suicidal adolescents: Comparison of CSF measures and fenfluramine challenge results.* Paper presented at the 38th annual meeting of the American Academy of Child and Adolescent Psychiatry, San Francisco, CA.

Grosz, D. E., Blackwood, N., Finkelstein, G., & Plutchik, R. (1991, April). *Correlates of suicide risk in adolescent inpatients.* Paper presented at the 24th annual meeting of the American Association of Suicidology, Boston, MA.

Häfner, H., & Schmidke, A. (1989). Do televised fictional suicide models produce suicides? In C. R. Pfeffer (Ed.), *Suicide among youth: Perspectives on risk and prevention* (pp. 117–142). Washington, DC: American Psychiatric Press.

Harkavy Friedman, J., Asnis, G., Boeck, M., & DiFiore, J. (1987). Prevalence of specific suicidal behaviors in a high school sample. *American Journal of Psychiatry, 144*(9), 1203–1206.

Hawton, K. (1986). *Suicide and attempted suicide among children and adolescents.* Newbury Park, CA: Sage.

Hawton, K. (1987). *Attempted suicide.* New York: Oxford University Press.

Hawton, K., O'Grady, J., Osborn, M., & Cole, D. (1982). Adolescents who take overdoses: Their characteristics, problems, and contacts with helping agencies. *British Journal of Psychiatry, 140,* 118–123.

Holden, R. R., Mendonca, J. D., & Serin, R. C. (1989). Suicide, hopelessness, and social desirability: A test of an interactive model. *Journal of Consulting and Clinical Psychology, 57,* 500–504.

Holinger, P. C. (1989). Epidemiological issues in youth suicide. In C. R. Pfeffer (Ed.), *Suicide among youth: Perspectives on risk and prevention* (pp. 41–62). Washington, DC: American Psychiatric Association.

Institute of Medicine. (1989). *Research on children and adolescents with mental, behavioral & developmental disorders.* Washington, DC: National Academy Press.

Isherwood, J., Adam, K. S., & Hornblow, A. R. (1982). Life event stress, psychosocial factors, suicide attempts, and auto-accident proclivity. *Journal of Psychosomatic Research, 26,* 371–383.

Jacobs, J. J. (1971). *Adolescent Suicide.* New York: John Wiley & Sons.

Jaffe, R. T., Offord, D. R., & Boyle, M. H. (1988). Ontario Child Health Study: Suicidal behavior in youth age 12–16 years. *American Journal of Psychiatry, 145,* 1420–1423.

Johnson, B., & Brent, D. (1991, October). *Personality and other predictors of suicidal behavior in adolescent inpatients.* Paper presented at the 38th annual meeting of the American Academy of Child and Adolescent Psychiatry, San Francisco, CA.

Kennedy, P., Kreitman, N., & Ovenstone, I. M. K. (1974). The prevalence of suicide and parasuicide ("attempted suicide") in Edinburgh. *British Journal of Psychiatry, 124,* 36–41.

Kety, S. (1986). Genetic factors in suicide. In A. Roy (Ed.), *Suicide* (pp. 41–45). Baltimore, MD: Williams & Wilkins.

King, C. A., Raskin, A., Gdowski, C. L., Butkus, M., & Opipari, L. (1990). Psychosocial factors associated with urban adolescent female suicide attempts. *Journal of the American Academy of Child and Adolescent Psychiatry, 29*(2), 289–294.

Kirkpatrick-Smith, K., Rich, A., Bonner, R., & Jans, F. (1989). Substance abuse and suicidal ideation among adolescents. In D. Lester (Ed.), *Suicide '89* (pp. 90–91). Denver, CO: American Association of Suicidology.

Kosky, R. (1983). Childhood suicidal behavior. *Journal of Child Psychology and Psychiatry, 24,* 457–468.

Kosky, R., Silburn, S., & Zubrick, S. (1986). Symptomatic depression and suicidal ideation: A comparative study with 628 children. *Journal of Nervous and Mental Diseases, 174,* 523–528.

Kuperman, S., Black, D. W., & Burnst, L. (1988). Excess suicide among formerly hospitalized child psychiatry patients. *Journal of Clinical Psychiatry, 49,* 88–93.

Lester, D. (1988). *The biochemical basis of suicide.* Springfield, IL: Charles C. Thomas.

Lester, D. (1992). Alcoholism and drug abuse. In R. W. Maris, A. L. Berman, J. T. Maltsberger, & R. I. Yufit (Eds.), *Assessment and prediction of suicide* (pp. 321–336). New York: The Guilford Press.

Lewinsohn, P. M. (1994). Psychosocial risk factors for future adolescent suicide attempts. *Journal of Consulting and Clinical Psychology, 62,* 297–305.

Lipschitz, D. S., Kaplan, M. L., & Asnis, G. M. (1994, May). *Characteristics of abuse in psychiatric outpatients.* Paper presented at the Annual Meeting of the American Psychiatric Association, Philadelphia, PA.

McBride, P. A., Brown, R. P., & DeMeo, M. (1987). Platelet 5-HT$_2$ receptors: Depression and suicide. *American Psychiatric Association New Research Abstracts,* NR157. Chicago, IL: American Psychiatric Association.

Mann, J. J., DeMeo, M. D., Keilp, J. G., & McBride, P. A. (1989). Biological correlates of suicidal behavior in youth. In C. R. Pfeffer (Ed.), *Suicide among youth: Perspectives on risk and prevention* (pp. 185–202). Washington, DC: American Psychiatric Press.

Meltzer, H. Y., & Lowy, M. T. (1989). The neuroendocrine system and suicide. In L. Davidson & M. Linnoila (Eds.), *Report of the Secretary's Task Force on Youth Suicide: (Vol. 2). Risk factors for youth suicide* (pp. 235–246). DHHS Pub. No. (ADM)89-1622. Washington, DC: U.S. Government Printing Office.

Motto, J. A. (1984). Suicide in male adolescents. In H. Sudak, A. B. Ford, & N. B. Rushforth (Eds.), *Suicide in the young* (pp. 227–244). Boston, MA: John Wright PSG.

Murphy, G. E., & Wetzel, R. D. (1980). Suicide risk by birth cohort in the United States, 1949–1974. *Archives of General Psychiatry, 37,* 519–523.

National Center for Health Statistics. (1991). *Vital statistics of the United States: Vol. 2. Mortality—Part A (for the years 1966–1988).* Washington, DC: U.S. Government Printing Office.

National Center for Health Statistics. (1992). *Monthly vital statistics report (vol. 40, no. 8).* Hyattsville, MD: U.S. Public Health Service.

Nelson, F. C. (1987). Evaluation of a youth suicide prevention program. *Adolescence, 88,* 813–825.

Nordström, P., Samuelsson, M., Åsberg, M., Träskman-Bendz, L., Åberg-Wistedt, A., Nordin, C., & Bertilsson, L. (1994). CSF 5-HIAA predicts suicide risk after attempted suicide. *Suicide and Life-Threatening Behavior, 24*(1), 1–9.

Orbach, I., & Bar-Joseph, H. (1993). The impact of a suicide prevention program for adolescents on suicidal tendencies, hopelessness, ego identity, and coping. *Suicide and Life-Threatening Behavior, 23*(2), 120–129.

Otto, O. (1972). Suicidal acts by children and adolescents: A follow-up study. *Acta Psychiatrica Scandinavia, 233*(suppl.), 7–123.

Paykel, E. S. (1989). Stress and life events. In L. Davidson & M. Linnoila (Eds.), *Report of the Secretary's Task Force on Youth Suicide: (Vol. 2). Risk factors for youth suicide* (pp. 110–130). DHHS Pub. No. (ADM)89-1622. Washington, DC: U.S. Government Printing Office.

Pfeffer, C. R. (1986). *The suicidal child.* New York: The Guilford Press.

Pfeffer, C. R. (1989a). Life stress and family risk factors for youth fatal and nonfatal suicidal behavior. In C. R. Pfeffer (Ed.), *Suicide among youth: Perspectives on risk and prevention* (pp. 143–164). Washington, DC: American Psychiatric Association.

Pfeffer, C. R. (1989b). Family characteristics and support systems as risk factors for youth suicidal behavior. In L. Davidson & M. Linnoila (Eds.), *Report of the Secretary's Task Force on Youth Suicide: (Vol. 2). Risk factors for youth suicide* (pp. 71–87). DHHS Pub. No. (ADM)89-1622. Washington, DC: U.S. Government Printing Office.

Pfeffer, C. R., Klerman, G. L., Hurt, S. W., Kakuma, T., Peskin, J. R., & Siefker, C. A. (1993). Suicidal children grow up: Rates and psychosocial risk factors for suicide attempts during follow-up. *Journal of the American Academy of Child and Adolescent Psychiatry, 32*(1), 106–113.

Pfeffer, C. R., Klerman, G. L., Hurt, S. W., Lesser, M., Peskin, J. R., & Siefker, C. A. (1991). Suicidal children grow up: Demographic and clinical risk factors for adolescent suicide attempts. *Journal of the American Academy of Child and Adolescent Psychiatry, 30*(4), 609–616.

Pfeffer, C. R., Lipkins, R., Plutchik, R., & Mizruchi, M. (1988). Normal children at risk for suicidal behavior: A two-year follow-up study. *Journal of the American Academy of Child and Adolescent Psychiatry, 27*, 202–209.

Pfeffer, C. R., Newcorn, J., Kaplan, G., Mizruchi, M. S., & Plutchik, R. (1988). Suicidal behavior in adolescent psychiatric inpatients. *Journal of the American Academy of Child and Adolescent Psychiatry, 27*, 357–361.

Phillips, D. P., Lesyna, K., & Paight, D. J. (1992). Suicide and the media. In R. W. Maris, A. L. Berman, J. T. Maltsberger, & R. I. Yufit (Eds.), *Assessment and prediction of suicide* (pp. 499–519). New York: The Guilford Press.

Phillips, D. P., & Paight, D. J. (1987). The impact of televised movies about suicide. *New England Journal of Medicine, 317*, 809–811.

Plutchik, R., & van Praag, H. M. (1986). The measurement of suicidality, aggressivity, and impulsivity. *Clinical Neuropharmacology, 4*(suppl. 9), 380–382.

Plutchik, R., van Praag, H. M., & Conte, H. R. (1989). Correlates of suicide and violence risk, III: A two-stage model of countervailing forces. *Psychiatry Research, 28*, 215–225.

Puig-Antich, J., Lukens, E., Davies, M., Goetz, D., Brennan-Quattrock, J., & Todak, G. (1985a). Psychosocial functioning in prepubertal major depressive disorders: I. Interpersonal relationships during the depressive episode. *Archives of General Psychiatry, 42*, 500–507.

Puig-Antich, J., Lukens, E., Davies, M., Goetz, D., Brennan-Quattrock, J., & Todak, G. (1985b). Psychosocial functioning in prepubertal major depressive disorders: II. Interpersonal relationships after sustained recovery from affective episode. *Archives of General Psychiatry, 42*, 511–517.

Rich, A., & Bonner, R. (1987). Concurrent validity of a stress vulnerability model of suicidal ideation and behavior: A follow-up study. *Suicide and Life-Threatening Behavior, 17*, 265–270.

Rich, C. L., Fowler, R. C., Fogarty, L. A., & Young, D. (1988). San Diego Suicide Study: III. Relationships between diagnoses and stressors. *Archives of General Psychiatry, 45,* 589–592.

Robbins, D. R., & Alessi, N. E. (1985). Depressive symptoms and suicidal behavior in adolescents. *American Journal of Psychiatry, 142,* 588–592.

Robins, L. N. (1978). Study of childhood predictors of adult antisocial behavior. *Psychological Medicine, 8,* 611–622.

Rolf, J., Masten, A. S., Cichetti, D., Neuchterlein, K., & Weintraub, S. (1990). *Risk and protective factors in developmental psychopathology.* New York: Cambridge University Press.

Rosenberg, M. L., Smith, J. C., Davidson, L. E., & Conn, J. M. (1987). The emergence of youth suicide: An epidemiologic analysis and public health perspective. *Annual Review of Public Health, 8,* 417–440.

Rotheram-Borus, M., Trautman, P., Dopkins, S., & Shrout, P. (1990). Cognitive styles and pleasant activities among female adolescent suicide attempters. *Journal of Consulting and Clinical Psychology, 58,* 554–561.

Roy, A. (1992). Genetics, biology, and the family. In R. W. Maris, A. L. Berman, J. T. Maltsberger, & R. I. Yufit (Eds.), *Assessment and prediction of suicide* (pp. 574–588). New York: The Guilford Press.

Roy, A. (1994). Recent biologic studies on suicide. *Suicide and Life-Threatening Behavior, 24*(1), 10–14.

Rubenstein, J., Heeren, T., Housman, D., Rubin, C., & Stechler, G. (1989). Suicide behavior in normal adolescents: Risk and protective factors. *American Journal of Orthopsychiatry, 59,* 59–71.

Rudd, M. D. (1990). An integrative model of suicidal ideation. *Suicide and Life-Threatening Behavior, 20*(1), 16–30.

Ryan, N. D., Puig-Antich, J., Rabinovich, H., Ambrosini, P., Robinson, D., Nelson, B., & Novacenko, H. (1988). Growth hormone response to desmethylimipramine in depressed and suicidal adolescents. *Journal of Affective Disorders, 15,* 323–337.

Sanderson, W. C., Friedman, T., Wetzler, S., Kaplan, M. L., & Asnis, G. M. (1992, November). Personality disorders in patients with major depression, panic disorder, and generalized anxiety disorder. Paper presented at the Annual Meeting of the Association for the Advancement of Behavioral Therapy, Boston, MA.

Sansonnet-Hayden, H., Haley, G., & Marriage, K. (1987). Sexual abuse and psychopathology in hospitalized adolescents. *Journal of the American Academy of Child and Adolescent Psychiatry, 26,* 753–757.

Schmidke, A., & Häfner, H. (1988). The Werther effect after television films: New evidence for an old hypothesis. *Psychological Medicine, 18,* 665–676.

Schotte, D., & Clum, G. (1982). Suicide ideation in a college population: A test of a model. *Journal of Consulting and Clinical Psychology, 55,* 49–54.

Schuckit, M. A., & Schuckit, J. J. (1989). Substance use and abuse: A risk factor in youth suicide. In L. Davidson & M. Linnoila (Eds.), *Report of the Secretary's Task Force on Youth Suicide: (Vol. 2). Risk factors for youth suicide* (pp. 172–183). DHHS Pub. No. (ADM)89-1622. Washington, DC: U.S. Government Printing Office.

Schulsinger, F., Kety, S., Rosenthal, D., & Wender, P. (1979). A family study of suicide. In M. Schou & E. Stromgren (Eds.), *Origin, prevention, and treatment of affective disorders* (pp. 277–287). London, UK: Academic Press.

Shaffer, D. (1974). Suicide in childhood and early adolescence. *Journal of Child Psychology and Psychiatry, 15,* 275–291.

Shaffer, D. (1988). The epidemiology of teen suicide: An examination of risk factors. *Journal of Clinical Psychiatry, 49,* 36–41.

Shaffer, D., Garland, A., & Bacon, K. (1989). Prevention issues in youth suicide. In D. Shaffer, I. Philips, & N. B. Enser (Eds.), *Prevention of mental disorders, alcohol, and other drug use in children and adolescents.* OSAP Prevention Monograph no. 2. Washington, DC: U.S. Department of Health and Human Services.

Shaffer, D., Garland, A., Gould, M., Fisher, P., & Trautman, P. (1988). Preventing teenage suicide: A critical review. *Journal of American Academy of Child Adolescence Psychiatry, 27*(6), 675–687.

Shaffer, D., Vieland, V., Garland, A., Rojas, M., Underwood, M., & Busner, C. (1990). Adolescent suicide attempters: Response to suicide prevention programs. *Journal of the American Medical Association, 264,* 3151–3155.

Shafii, M., Carrigan, S., Whittinghill, L., & Derrick, A. (1985). Psychological autopsy of completed suicide in children and adolescents. *American Journal of Psychiatry, 142,* 1061–1064.

Smith, J. C., Mercy, J. A., & Rosenberg, M. L. (1986). Suicide and homicide among Hispanics in the Southwest. *Public Health Reports, 101,* 265–270.

Smith, K., & Crawford, S. (1986). Suicidal behavior among normal high school students. *Suicide and Life-Threatening Behavior, 16,* 313–325.

Solomon, M. I., & Hellon, C. P. (1980). Suicide and age in Alberta, Canada, 1951–1977. *Archives of General Psychiatry, 37,* 511–513.

Sorenson, S. B., & Golding, J. M. (1988). Suicide ideation and attempts in Hispanics and non-Hispanic whites: Demographic and psychiatric disorder issues. *Suicide and Life-Threatening Behavior, 18,* 205–218.

Spirito, A., Overholser, J., Ashworth, S., Morgan, J., & Benedict-Drew, C. (1988). Evaluation of a suicide awareness curriculum for high school students. *Journal of the American Academy of Child and Adolescent Psychiatry, 27*(6), 705–711.

Stack, S. (1987). Celebrities and suicide: A taxonomy and analysis, 1948–1983. *American Sociological Review, 52,* 401–412.

Stack, S. (1993). The media and suicide: A nonadditive model, 1968–1980. *Suicide and Life-Threatening Behavior, 23*(1), 63–66.

Stack, S., Gundlach, J., & Reeves, J. (1994). The heavy metal subculture and suicide. *Suicide and Life-Threatening Behavior, 24*(1), 15–23.

Stanley, E. J., & Barter, J. T. (1970). Adolescent suicidal behavior. *American Journal of Orthopsychiatry, 40,* 87–96.

Stanley, M. (1989). Post mortem studies of suicide. In L. Davidson & M. Linnoila (Eds.), *Report of the Secretary's Task Force on Youth Suicide: (Vol. 2). Risk factors for youth suicide* (pp. 213–234). DHHS Pub. No. (ADM)89-1622. Washington, DC: U.S. Government Printing Office.

Swanson, J. W., Linskey, A. O., Quintero-Salinas, R., Pumariega, A. J., & Holzer, C. E. (1992). A binational school survey of depressive symptoms, drug use, and suicidal ideation. *Journal of the American Academy of Child and Adolescent Psychiatry, 31,* 669–678.

Tischler, C., McKenry, P., & Morgan, K. (1981). Adolescent suicide attempts: Some significant factors. *Suicide and Life-Threatening Behavior, 11,* 86–92.

Topol, P., & Reznikoff, M. (1982). Perceived peer and family relationships, hopelessness, and locus of control as factors in adolescent suicide attempts. *Suicide and Life-Threatening Behavior, 12,* 141–150.

van Praag, H. M., Asnis, G. M., Kahn, R. S., Brown, S. L., Korn, M., Harkavy Friedman, J. M., & Wetzler, S. (1990). Nosological tunnel vision in biological psychiatry. *Annals of the New York Academy of Sciences, 600,* 501–510.

Vega, W. A., Gil, A., Warheit, G., Apospori, E., & Zimmerman, R. (1993). The relationship of drug use to suicide ideation and attempts among African American, Hispanic, and White Non-Hispanic male adolescents. *Suicide and Life-Threatening Behavior, 23*(2), 110–119.

Welner, A., Welner Z., & Fishman, R. (1979). Psychiatric inpatients: Eight- to ten-year follow-up. *Archives of General Psychiatry, 36,* 689–700.

Wetzel, R. D., Margulies, T., Davis, R., & Karam, E. (1980). Hopelessness, depression, and suicide intent. *Journal of Clinical Psychiatry, 41,* 159–160.

Yang, B., & Clum, G. A. (1994). Life stress, social support, and problem-solving skills predictive of depressive symptoms, hopelessness, and suicide ideation in an Asian student population: A test of a model. *Suicide and Life-Threatening Behavior, 24*(2), 127–139.

Zimmerman, J. K., & Morledge, J. (1992). *Prevalence of specific suicidal behaviors in a high school sample: A replication and extension.* Unpublished manuscript.

PART II
Diagnosis, Assessment, and Crisis Intervention

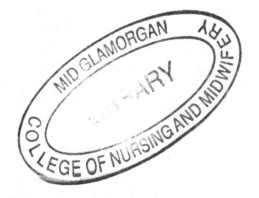

3

Assessment and Prediction of Suicide Risk in Adolescents

ANTOON A. LEENAARS AND
DAVID LESTER

No one can predict suicide perfectly. The suicidal person's poverty of thought is regrettably all too often symbiotically mimicked by some to a reductionistic way to predict it. In both cases there is no perfect solution but perhaps a shared state of mind: mental constriction. Suicide prediction is complex, especially in the assessment and prediction of suicide in young people. "The teenager is suicidal" is a prediction. How do we make such a prediction? If we are to answer this question, we should not see assessment and prediction as separate from *understanding*. In fact, we will argue that understanding is still the only key that allows us to approximate sound—not perfect—prediction.

One reason, if not the reason, why it is so difficult to predict suicide is that usually we deal only with the end result. With other mental health issues, we are not faced with this obstacle. For example, if we wish to predict a learning disability, we can make some hypotheses, investigate them, refine them, and so forth. In suicide, obviously, we cannot do this. The search for *the* test or *the* clue of predicting a behavior as complex as suicide is a wishful fancy. There is no *one* test. There is no *one* clue.

Clinicians wishing to understand and predict any behavior, in fact, have long ago abandoned the notion of using one instrument. To use just one test is, in fact, to regress to the days of phrenology, when it was believed that if we could find the right bump on a person's head we would know his or her personality, IQ, and the like—and, we assume, his or her suicidal tendencies. Even the earliest use of standardized tests in mental health (e.g., Galton's questionnaire methods, Cattell's mental tests, Binet's test) was criticized as needing to address this

problem (Anastasi, 1982). In response to the recognition of such sim-
plification, clinicians developed a wide-ranging approach (e.g., tests,
interview, observation, third-person consultations, use of personal
documents) and acknowledged the need to use their clinical judgment
to understand the observations. To predict suicide, we believe that we
must adopt such a comprehensive approach, or we will be forever
searching for the "bump" that will tell all. An example of such an approach was recently presented (Leenaars, 1992), showing how suicide
notes can be a guide to prediction.

Given all this, and if the reader has any optimism left, let us offer
here a few signposts that may illuminate the quest.

Case Example

Bruce, a nearly 16-year-old male, was referred to an outpatient psychiatric facility. Bruce presented himself as a very defensive, aggressive individual. He was strikingly angry at the world. He was referred by the
local school system after being suspended. It is noteworthy that Bruce
had been previously referred for assistance since grade 2 and was now in
grade 9. His divorced mother had refused all such referrals in the past.
The only reason for accepting the referral this time was because the
school system had stated that unless Bruce got help, they could not cope
with his behavior. The underlying reason, however, was that Bruce was
exhibiting similar behavior at home for the first time.

At the time of the referral, Bruce was extremely oppositional and deviant. He would verbally assault any teacher who made the slightest request, which he experienced invariably as a provocation. Being
overactive, almost hyperactive, he was constantly out of his seat. This
and other disruptions would result in classroom conflict and the ever-
present trip to the office. Here the situation would escalate. "Fuck off"
became Bruce's every second phrase.

Bruce's parents separated when Bruce was in grade 2. According to
the mother, his father was an alcoholic. The father, on the other hand,
denied this, stating that he had been perplexed about having been kicked
out of the house one day. He described his ex-wife as a rejecting, ambivalent, moody person. Little is known about the actual history. The mother
was excessively evasive when questioned. The father reported one episode of depression, resulting in hospitalization. Neither parent knew of
any other psychiatric disorder in the extended family.

Bruce had three older brothers. Their history was equally problematic. School problems had occurred. Legal conflicts were frequent. Bruce

was labeled as "the baby" in the family, constantly striving to be like his brothers. Yet his mother needed him to be with her; often he was her only companion at night and on outings.

Psychological testing had been completed by the school system before the referral for treatment. The background information in the report included the following: Bruce had experienced early success in school, being well liked by his female teachers. In grade 3, his performance worsened. A referral for a mental health assessment at that time was not followed up by the mother. Vision testing suggested that he was mildly myopic. There were no medical/physical illnesses beyond the common ones of childhood.

Test results from the school included information about current intellectual and academic functioning. Based on his performance on the Wechsler Intelligence Scale for Children-Revised (WISC-R [Wechsler, 1974]), Bruce's overall intellectual functioning fell within the Average range (Full Scale IQ of 99), with no significant difference between verbal-language areas (Verbal IQ of 101) and visual-spatial areas (Performance IQ of 92). His true Full Scale IQ has a likelihood of falling in the 94–104 range (Kaufman, 1979). Considerable variation was noted in WISC-R subtests; Bruce especially had difficulties in attention, mental arithmetic, range of general factual information, and speed and accuracy at completing written tasks. A relative strength was noted in holistic thinking.

Bruce's basic academic skills, as measured by the Wide Range Achievement Test-Revised (WRAT-R [Jastak & Wilkinson, 1984]), was significantly discrepant from his WISC-R IQ. Reading, spelling, and arithmetic were deficient, generally at a grade 2 to 3 level. Auditory processing problems were identified from his performance in reading and spelling. A referral for neuropsychological testing to confirm a hypothesis of a learning disability was made but never followed. A recommendation also was made that Bruce initiate individual long-term psychotherapy, which resulted in his referral to the outpatient service.

A DEVELOPMENTAL PERSPECTIVE

To understand any young person, a developmental view is essential. This is as true in suicide as in other aspects of mental health. There are various perspectives on development, and we can make only a few points here. Erik Erikson's model (Erikson, 1963, 1964, 1968) continues to be useful in this endeavor. An infant's first task is the development of "trust versus mistrust" within relationships, especially with the mother. At about age two, the child begins to develop "autonomy versus shame and doubt," followed by "initiative versus guilt" from the ages of four to six. At around six, the period in which Bruce's first trouble appeared, the child's development centers around "industry versus inferiority." Indeed, inferiority marked Bruce's years after grade 2. He did not do well in school and his work was not satisfying. The breakup of the family left Bruce traumatized. His mother later reported that she wondered if Bruce ever felt equal to his classmates.

The teen years, ages 12 to 18, are marked by the integration of the past into a new configuration. The person needs to learn to cope with impulses, aptitudes, and social demands. The adolescent searches for a sense of identity. Limitations (e.g., having been abused, having a brain dysfunction) strongly affect this process. Doubts about oneself, such as one's acceptance by others, can be unbearably painful. Often, as with Bruce, these years become a period of floundering and insecurity, with such symptoms as isolation, emptiness, anxiety, and indecisiveness developing. Faced with inner turmoil and/or outer distress, the adolescent becomes unable to meet demands, sometimes even resisting them, and an identity confusion evolves. A false or fragile sense of self emerges, being strongly adhered to for any sense of "I"; this was certainly the case for Bruce.

There are other theoretical perspectives: Classics in the field are Blos (1979), Esman (1975), Anna Freud (1965), and Laufer (1975). Anyone wishing to work with teenagers must have an a priori understanding of these views before attempting to understand suicide. A developmental perspective is a prolegomenon to any assessment and prediction of adolescent suicide.

Next, and not separate from a developmental perspective, is the need for a schematic profile to assess an adolescent. Anna Freud's developmental profile offers one such example (Eissler, Freud, Kris, & Salmit, 1977). Maltsberger (1992) recently has provided an overview for schematic formulation in suicide, highlighting personal factors, exterior factors, and mental state phenomena. To discuss this in detail would be beyond the scope of this chapter, and we can only encourage the reader to seek out a model with which he or she becomes familiar and comfortable.

PREDICTION VERSUS ASSESSMENT

In the 1960s and 1970s, there was a focus on the prediction of suicide, and suicidologists believed that eventually it would be possible to predict which individuals out of a population ultimately would complete suicide (Beck, Resnik, & Lettieri, 1974). However, it was soon realized that the statistical rarity of suicide and the imperfection of the prediction instruments led to an enormously large number of false positives; so many, in fact, that the prediction instruments were of little use to clinicians or to those planning suicide prevention services.

In the 1980s and 1990s, the focus shifted to assessment (Maltsberger, 1992). That is, rather than trying to predict the future occurrence of suicide, the intent was to assess potentially suicidal people in a more general sense, taking into account all of their life experiences and psychological characteristics that are relevant to future suicidal behavior. Indeed, it is our belief that prediction and assessment are mutual processes and any separation is an artificial one. They are not separate categories.

LETHALITY AND PERTURBATION

In assessing suicide in adolescents, we need to be aware of behaviors that are potentially predictive of suicide. Unfortunately, there is no such definitive behavior. Suicide is a multidimensional malaise (Leenaars, 1988a; Shneidman, 1985). Nevertheless, two preliminary concepts that may be helpful are *lethality* and *perturbation*. Lethality refers to the probability of a person killing him- or herself, and on quantification scales ranges from low to moderate to high. It is a psychological state of mind (although the term also is used in the field as referring to the likelihood that a suicide attempt will result in death). Perturbation refers to subjective distress, and also can be rated from low to moderate to high. Both have to be evaluated. It is important to note that one can be perturbed and not suicidal. Lethality kills, not perturbation. Perturbation often is relatively easy to evaluate; lethality is not. Lethality is best assessed by a professional with experience in that area. The concepts of lethality and perturbation are, thus, critical in one's professional assessment and prediction.

TESTS TO PREDICT SUICIDE

Over the last few decades, numerous attempts at constructing tests for suicide prediction and related phenomena have been made. Probably one of the best tests is Shneidman's (1973) simple measure (or more accurately, question): "During the last 24 hours, I felt my chances of actually killing myself (committing suicide and ending my life) were: Absent, very low, low medium, fifty-fifty, high medium, very high, extra high (came very close to actually killing myself)" (p. 384). Generally, clinical experience has shown that many patients can predict their own suicide risk (and often are relieved to find someone willing to talk about their ominous prediction).

Unfortunately, in our case example, Bruce was little inclined to answer such questions. He denied any problem, projecting all the problems on the school, especially on Miss Jones, the vice-principal at the school, in charge of discipline. He described her as "a bitch." When asked about himself, he said, "It's all bullshit." When asked what he meant, he just repeated this statement. Again, he was asked, "What is the 'it'?" He responded that his life, school, and family were "bullshit," adding "It's just boring." He especially focused on school, seeing no hope. He responded to Schneidman's suicide question with: "Do I have any meaning?"

Are there any tests that could help us predict Bruce's suicide risk? Recently, due to awareness of the phenomenon of suicide in youth, the National Institutes of Mental Health (NIMH) organized a think tank in the assessment of suicidal behavior in adolescents (Lewinsohn, Garrison, Langhinrichsen, & Marsteller, 1989). This group found that there were inherent difficulties, as we noted, in the assessment of suicidal behavior. Suicide is not a psychopathological entity in the fourth edition of the *Diagnostic and Statistical Manual of Mental Disorders* (DSM-IV) (American Psychiatric Association, 1994). Within this frame, they reviewed all available assessment instruments used to study suicidal behavior in adolescents. The conclusion: *Few, if any, are useful.* The NIMH group found numerous problems in the instruments; for example, ambiguity of the purpose of the instrument, insufficient attention to validity, the lack of discrimination between suicide risk and other forms of self-destructive behavior, and the lack of theoretical models. Our own impression agrees to date: Each of these tests, by itself, has little utility. However, within the context of the clinician's skill, they may be useful. The reader is urged to read a summary of this work by Garrison, Lewinsohn, Marsteller, Langhinrichsen, and Lann (1991).

Despite this state of affairs, the NIMH group did isolate two instruments that had some potential in predicting suicide risk, (i.e., the intent to kill oneself): the Beck Suicide Intent Scale and the Lethality of Suicide Attempt Rating Scale.

Beck Suicide Intent Scale (BSIS)

This instrument was developed by Aaron T. Beck. (See Beck, Kovacs, & Weissman, 1979; Steer & Beck, 1988.) It is a semistructured interview administered by a trained clinician. The BSIS describes a person's behavior and environmental circumstances and the person's attitudes, thoughts, and feelings about suicide. There are reliability and validity data. (See Lewinsohn et al., 1989.) The NIMH group concluded, and we concur, that it is "an important instrument."

Lethality of Suicide Attempt Rating Scale (LSARS)

This scale was developed by Kim Smith and his colleagues. (See Smith, Conroy, & Ehler, 1984.) It measures the degree of lethality of intent. Psychometric data are available. The NIMH group concluded that the scale has potential, and we echo this view from our clinical experience. Yet its use with adolescents has not been reported. Therefore, if one wishes to use such scales, we recommend that both the BSIS and the LSARS be used together.

Upon reconstruction of notes, Bruce's evaluation on both the Beck and Smith scales would suggest low lethality at intake.

Maltsberger (1992) recently reviewed the area of assessment and prediction, concluding that the richness and diversity of suicidal behavior could not be reduced to a single, definitive test. In part, we believe that the attempt to search for *the* test is also reflective of the misconception of being test-focused as opposed to person-focused (Kral, 1992). It is the person who is suicidal. Only by understanding the person can one assess and predict suicide.

There are, of course, other tests that have utility in understanding the person who is at risk for suicide. The Rorschach (Rorschach, 1942/ 1981), Thematic Apperception Test (Murray, 1943), and Minnesota Multiphasic Personality Inventory (REF) are just a few that may be used in an assessment battery, although not as a single test (Eyman & Eyman, 1992; Leenaars, 1992). There also are scales regarding specific associated variables such as depression (Beck & Steer, 1987;

Kovacs, 1985; Reynolds, 1986; Steer & Beck, 1988), hopelessness (Beck, Weissman, Lester, & Trexler, 1974; Kazdin, Rodgas, & Colbus, 1986), and life events (Holmes & Rahe, 1967; Johnson & Mc-Cutcheon, 1980; Sarason, Johnson, & Siegel, 1978). However, more comprehensive instruments such as the Thematic Guide for Suicide Prediction (TGSP—Leenaars, 1992) may prove to be more useful in the future than these specific measures. It should be clear, however, that none of these tests should be used as a single test and that a clinician may have little utility for them individually.

It also should be noted that there is often a dispute as to the relative merits of the clinical intuition of a mental health professional about a patient's suicidal potential versus the numerical, precise scores from objective tests. Lester (1974) has pointed out that these two approaches are not antagonistic. Not only can clinical intuition be included in the overall assessment of a patient, but if either intuition or objective psychological tests indicate a potential for suicidal behavior, the clinician should proceed with caution with the patient.

UNDERSTANDING SUICIDE BY ASSESSMENT AND PREDICTION

If one attempts to understand suicide, one becomes aware over time of its enormous complexity. Suicide can be defined as an event with biological, psychological, interpersonal, situational, sociological, cultural, and philosophical/existential components. Each can be an avenue to assessment. From our clinical experience, we offer a few observations on the event with the understanding that these are not exhaustive. The following ideas are only a few signposts from suicidology on the quest for prediction of suicide.

Definition

Defining suicide is a complex endeavor in itself. Shneidman (1985) has provided the following definition: "Currently in the Western world, suicide is a conscious act of self-induced annihilation, best understood as a multidimensional malaise in a needful individual who defines an issue for which suicide is perceived as the best solution" (p. 203).

Pfeffer (1986) has suggested that the definition of suicide needs to be clarified somewhat for youth. She has provided the following comment:

It is not necessary for a child to have an understanding of the finality of death but it is necessary to have a concept of death, regardless of how idiosyncratic it may be. Therefore, suicidal behavior in children can be defined as self-destructive behavior that has the intent to seriously damage oneself or cause death. (P. 14)

For assessment, one should keep Shneidman's definition in the foreground with Pfeffer's clarification always in mind with youth.

Concept of Death

Do children and adolescents understand death? Pfeffer's research (Pfeffer, 1986) suggests that the answer is yes, although ideas of death differ depending on the age of the person. Young children (approximately at age seven) see death as temporary; further, everything—animate and inanimate as well—is alive and vulnerable to death. Children around ten years of age see death as personified and temporary; an outside agent causes death. By the time a child—a young adolescent—is approximately 13 years old, he or she sees death as final: Internal biological processes cause death. Yet even older adolescents may misunderstand or ignore the finality of death. Bruce's idea of life was that it was "meaningless"; he saw no benefit in it. He would state, "What's the use; I'll only end up in a factory," adding his favorite line: "It's all bullshit." Bruce had his own pessimistic understanding of life, but did he understand the finitude of death?

Previous Attempts

Although it is obvious that one has to "attempt" suicide in order to commit it, it is equally clear that the event of "attempting suicide" need not have death as its objective. It is useful to think of the "attempter" (now often referred to as a parasuicide) and the "completer" as two sets of overlapping populations: (1) a group of those who attempt suicide, a few of whom go on to commit it; and (2) a group of those who commit suicide, some of whom previously attempted it. A good deal has to do with the lethality of the event. The ratio between suicide attempts and completions in the general population is about eight to one—one committed suicide for every eight attempts (Shneidman, 1985); however, in teenagers some studies report a rate of 50 to 1, even 100 to 1 (Berman & Jobes, 1991).

A previous attempt is a good indicator of risk for future attempts, especially if no assistance is obtained after the first attempt. However, not all previous attempters go on to kill themselves; about 15 percent do so, versus 1.5 percent for the general population (Lester, 1992). However, all too frequently such behavior is not taken seriously. Bruce was not an attempter when he began treatment.

Verbal Statements

As with suicidal behavior, the attitude toward individuals making verbal threats is too frequently negative. Such statements are seen as being made just for attention. This results in dismissing or ignoring the behavior of a person who is genuinely perturbed and potentially suicidal. The important question is: "Why this way of getting attention when there are so many other constructive ways?"

Examples of verbal statements from young people are the following: "I'm going to kill myself" or "I want to die." Both are very direct. Other more indirect examples are the following: "I am going to see my (deceased) mother" or "I know that I'll die at an early age." Bruce's expressions—"It's all meaningless" and "What's the use?"—may be examples of such indirect statements.

Cognitive Clues

The single most frequent state of mind of the suicidal person is *constriction*. There is a tunnel vision, a narrowing of the range of perception or opinions or options that occur to the mind. Frequently the person uses words such as "only," "always," "never," and "forever." Examples from young people are the following: "No one will ever love me. Only Mom loved me"; "John was the only one who loved me"; "Dad will always be that way"; and "Either I'll kill my brother or myself." Bruce's vocabulary was full of "all," "never," "more," and so on. His mind was constricted; he was guarded and rigid. About his future, he only saw more "bullshit." He stated: "It will never change," adding with a musical tone, "Life is just a one-way ticket."

Sudden Behavioral Changes

Changes in behavior also are suspect. Both the outgoing individual who suddenly becomes withdrawn and isolated and the normally reserved individual who begins to take risks and seek thrills may be at risk. Such changes are of particular concern when a precipitating painful event is apparent. Changes in school performance, such as sudden failure, may be important clues. Making final arrangements, such as giving away a music collection, a favorite watch, or other possessions, may be ominous and often not responded to by the recipient; the recipient is simply too pleased to get the "gift." A sudden preoccupation with death, such as reading and talking about it excessively, also may be a clue.

A marker of Bruce's personality was his erratic behavior. His mood swings were extreme. One never knew what to expect; little things would trigger behavioral change. Was it biological? Was he showing early signs of a manic-depressive illness or borderline features? Signs such as giving things away (he never gave away anything) and preoccupations did not occur; yet, why the erratic behavior?

Depression

First and foremost, it must be understood that not all suicidal youth are depressed and that not all depressed youth are suicidal. Depression and suicide are *not* equivalent. Yet Pfeffer (1986) has noted that depression sometimes distinguishes suicidal adolescents from nonsuicidal groups. Depression can be noted in mood and behavior (ranging from hesitancy in social contacts and feeling dejected to isolation, remoteness, and serious disturbance of appetite and sleep); verbal expression (ranging from talk about being disappointed, excluded, blamed, and so on, to talk of suicide, being killed, abandoned, helpless); and thought (ranging from feeling disappointed and thinking one is excluded, mistreated, and the like, to thoughts of suicide, self-mutilation, and preoccupation with the loss of a significant person). Behaviors such as excessive aggressiveness, sleep disturbance, change in school performance, decreased socialization, somatic complaints, loss of energy, and unusual change in appetite and weight have all been associated with depression (Pfeffer, 1986).

However, not all depression is overt. Teenagers often exhibit what has been termed "masked depression" (Leenaars & Wenckstern, 1991). Anorexia, promiscuity, and drug abuse, for example, have been associated with depression (Berman & Jobes, 1991). In Bruce's case, he was certainly depressed, as evidenced in pessimistic thoughts, irritable and angry mood, poor socialization and school performance, and so on. Historical data suggested that this had been true for years.

It is important to remember, however, that depression does not equal suicide in a simple one-to-one fashion. Most suicides experience *unbearable pain,* but not necessarily depression (Shneidman, 1985). The unbearable emotion might be hostility, despair, shame, guilt, dependency, hopelessness, and/or helplessness. What is critical is that the emotion—pain—is unbearable. In teenagers, this pain often is expressed in anger. In fact, very angry and hostile adolescents sometimes may be more at risk for suicide than adolescents exhibiting more traditional signs of depression. Bruce's anger was pronounced; it was expressed uncontrollably, resulting, for example, in his being banned from the local recreation facility. He was not only aggressive with other youth, but with staff as well. His ever-present "fuck you" only added to his isolation. He could not tolerate his emotions when among others.

Learning Disabilities

The importance of brain dysfunction in children and its relation to learning disabilities is well documented (Rourke, Young, & Leenaars, 1989). The relation of brain dysfunction to socioemotional problems is, however, a more neglected topic in the literature, despite an apparent correlation with suicidality. Peck (1985) has observed that, although about 5 percent of children are diagnosed as learning disabled in the general population, in a sample of suicidal youngsters, 50 percent had been so labeled. He noted:

> It is clear that learning disabled youngsters may suffer from loss of esteem, and in those cases where youngsters experience both pressure from parents to be "normal" and pressure from peers deriding their disability, their feelings of frustrations and hurt may be so great as to place a very young child in an at-risk category for suicide. (P. 116)

Although Peck's observations are important for understanding the development of suicidal behavior, he does not take note of the additional point that there are particular subtypes of learning disabilities and that these different subtypes may result in different levels of risk. Different patterns of cerebral dysfunction and their resulting learning disabilities render a teenager at risk for different types of socioemotional disturbances. There are three major subgroups

(Rourke & Fisk, 1981; Rourke, Young, & Leenaars, 1989). The first group has a right brain dysfunction. These adolescents are prone to learning problems with nonverbal, visual information. These adolescents may show the following socioemotional problems: not paying attention to visual objects including other people in the classroom, playground, and so on; rarely expressing emotions appropriately in their facial expressions; having a voice that can be expressionless; being very talkative; talking to self; having flow problems in their speech; and being awkward socially. The second group has a left brain dysfunction. These adolescents are prone to learning problems with verbal information. They may show the following socioemotional problems: rarely initiating conversations; having problems paying attention, for example, in conversation; being brief and often concrete in their remarks; often stating "I don't know" to questions; and being impulsive, not thinking before they act. The third group has both left and right brain dysfunction and exhibits a conglomerate of symptoms.

Often more specific cerebral deficits render people at risk for other specific problems such as in planning, sequencing social events, and the like. Although further empirical studies need to be conducted in the neuropsychology of youth suicides, these observations clearly warrant attention. Indeed, Rourke, Young, and Leenaars (1989) have shown that one possible adolescent (and adult) outcome of childhood central processing deficiencies is suicidal behavior. They have suggested that it is especially the first pattern (associated with right brain dysfunction) that predisposes those afflicted to adolescent (and adult) suicide risk.

Having said all that, Bruce was, as hypothesized, learning disabled, but it was not related to a right brain dysfunction; his disability was more reflective of a disability of left hemispheric origin. He had problems in paying attention. He was very explosive. He rarely initiated conversation, waiting for others to ask questions. In treatment, one had to modify one's language to get him to understand.

When Bruce was confronted with the results of the psychological testing, he said, "I don't give a fuck." He suggested that he did not try, although the examiner remarked that Bruce tried on most tests. Bruce seemed to be generally unaware and not accepting of his deficits, blaming the school for his problems. This characteristic is not unusual in people with left brain dysfunctions.

Physical Disabilities and Illness

We would be remiss if we did not note the importance of physical problems in suicidal behavior in some youth. Physical illness interacts with an individual's emotional functioning; indeed, some illnesses even directly affect one's emotions. Some physical illnesses that have been associated, according to Barraclough (1986), with suicidal behavior (although he does not differentiate for what age) are anorexia, bulimia, diabetes, epilepsy, traumatic brain injury, and muscular dystrophia. Among individuals with physical disabilities who are at risk are those with limb amputations or spinal injuries resulting in quadriplegia. In addition, individuals with terminal illness such as AIDS (often at the early stages of this disease) appear to be at high risk (Fryer, 1986; Marzuk, 1989). We also recall a case of a young male who had a genital malformation, which contributed significantly to his suicidal solution. Even acne may be too much to bear in some vulnerable individuals. However, it is important to realize that not all such youth are suicidal and that empirical study regarding the relationship between illness and suicide in adolescents is urgently needed. In Bruce's case, no physical disabilities or illness was present.

Specific Environmental Precipitating Events

A current popular formulation regarding suicide is that suicide is simply due to an external event; for example, a rejection, the influence of the music of a pop singer, whatever. This is a myth. Nevertheless, it is true that precipitating events (e.g., deprivation of love, sexual abuse, death of parent, divorce, rejection) do occur in the suicides of adolescents (Pfeffer, 1986), although often it is difficult to attribute the act to a single precipitant. We are here reminded of a clinical example. A 16-year-old teenager was found dead in a car, having died of carbon monoxide poisoning. People were perplexed: "Why did this young person from an upper-middle-class family kill himself?" The parents found out that his girlfriend rejected him the day of his suicide. Some thought that was *the* reason. When a young person gets rejected and is so in love, he may kill himself. A few friends and his teachers knew that he had been having problems in school. They thought *that* was the reason. A few others knew that his father was an alcoholic and abusive. *That* was the reason for them. His doctor knew that he had been adopted and had been upset recently about that. She knew *the* real reason. And others knew . . .

Shneidman (1985) maintained that the common factor in suicide is not the precipitating event but *lifelong coping patterns.* Even in youth, one can see a continuity despite developmental changes. Adolescents who kill themselves have experienced a steady toll of threat, stress, failure, challenge, and loss that gradually undermined their adjustment process. Their history is critical to their suicidal solution (Leenaars, 1988a).

The event that marked Bruce's decline in functioning was his transfer to a new school, geared for more vocational education. After Bruce had been seen for psychotherapy for several weeks, an academic review with Miss Jones, the vice-principal at his school, was undertaken. As a result of this review, Bruce was placed in a new school, becoming, in his word, "pissed." He stated that the school was for "tards." He attacked his therapist, his mother, the teachers, everyone. He threatened the therapist, stating that the therapist was supposed to help him and was not doing so. He denied any academic problems. His behavior led to expulsion from a recreation center and eventually from the new school. It was not that Bruce's behavior was new; rather, he showed the same behavior as in his old school, only now it became more generalized. He was especially angry at his mother. Why had she sent—abandoned—him to that school? The home situation deteriorated. Questions arose at this time about drug and alcohol use. Despite denial, Bruce's behavior was clearly reflective of it. He was often drunk at home. His moods began to fluctuate even more extremely. But was he more at risk for suicide?

Life-Threatening Behavior

We recall a 17-year-old teenager who died in a single-car accident on an isolated road after having had several similar accidents following his mother's death. *Self-destructiveness is not rare in adolescence.* Often alcoholism, drug addiction, mismanagement of medical treatment, and auto accidents can be seen in this light. Farberow (1980) has referred to this as "the many faces of suicide." Here are a number of questions related to self-destructive behavior:

- Why did a teenager play with the gun, knowing it was loaded?
- Why did a teenager drive so fast on a wet, slippery road when he knew for the last three months how bad his brakes were?

• Why did a person, knowing how cocaine could affect her, get hooked?

We are not suggesting that these young people intentionally wanted to die; yet their behavior made them "as good as dead." Bruce's behavior was self-destructive, and after the transfer to the new school, it became even more so. Drinking increased. He often lashed out aggressively at older males, inviting conflict. Suspicion arose about his criminal involvement. During one of his sessions with his therapist, Bruce said, "The only way for me to make money is steal it." He often had money the source of which could not be explained. The police became more and more involved in the case.

Suicide Notes

Like previous attempts and verbal statements, notes about suicide are important clues (Leenaars, 1988a). However, they are often read but not attended to by the reader. Although most adolescents who kill themselves do not leave a suicide note, some teenagers do so. Artwork, diaries, music, and other personal documents can be seen as similar expressive behaviors. We remember one suicide note stating "I finally completed something I've always wanted to do. I removed the guilt from every person . . . P.S.: Happy Father's Day."

Bruce wrote no note—in fact, he rarely wrote anything. Remember that his reading and spelling were at a grade 2 to 3 level. Yet perhaps his musical interests can be seen as a similar thematic expression. He loved the group Suicidal Tendencies. He often would isolate himself at home listening to his tapes over and over. After the expulsion from the recreational facility, this became even more of a preoccupation. He had few friends. He commented that "no one" understood him, adding again "It's all bullshit." His favorite song lyrics told of being alone, distraught, and wishing to "end it."

He once brought those lines in to the therapist, stating "This is me," adding that the title of the song was "Kill Yourself" by the group Storm Troopers of Death. The music, his "Doc's" boots, his clothes, and so on, were all expressions of his adherence to an antisocial and self-destructive subculture.

Suicidal Youth and Their Families

A review of the literature (e.g., Berman & Jobes, 1991; Corder & Haizlip, 1984; Corder, Parker, & Corder, 1974; Leenaars, 1988b;

Leenaars & Wenckstern, 1991; Maris, 1985; Pfeffer, 1981a, 1981b, 1986; Seiden, 1984; and Toolan, 1981) suggests that the family system and its functioning is a central factor associated with suicide and suicidal behavior in adolescents, although by no means do all families of suicidal adolescents display a characteristic pattern of dysfunction. (It is important to recall that there are no universals in suicide.) Based on a review of the previous references, here are a few common observations regarding suicidal adolescents and their families.

1. There is, at times, a lack of generational boundaries in suicidal families. There is an insufficient separation of the parent from his or her family of origin. For example, often grandparents take over the parenting role.

2. The family system is often inflexible. Denial, secretiveness, and especially a *lack of communication* are seen in the family. Any change is seen as a threat to the survival of the family. In response to the pressure implicit in this resistance to change, one 15-year-old boy once reported to us, "If I kill myself, then my dad will *have* to change." Additionally, such families have stringent discipline patterns and limit setting; for example, in some cases, love affairs are stopped by parents, even in eighteen-year-old youngsters. This inflexibility in the family system restricts the individual in the critical, age-appropriate process of identity development.

3. At times, there is a symbiotic parent-child relationship. A parent, usually the mother, is too attached to the youth. Not only is such a relationship disturbing, but the parent also does not provide the emotional protection and support that a parent usually provides intuitively to a youth as he or she grows. Sometimes the parent treats the youth as an "adult." One such teenager tried to break this bond by attempting to kill herself in her mother's prized car, while another—a straight A student—intentionally obtained a B, resulting in a parental conflict and a suicide attempt by the youth. Additionally, we have noted repeatedly in children that if a symbiotically enmeshed parent dies, the adolescent may commit suicide to be magically reunited with that parent.

4. Long-term disorganization (malfunctioning) has been noted in families of suicidal adolescents; for example, maternal or paternal absence, divorce, alcoholism, mental illness. In teenage girls (and boys) there is a very high rate of incest, compared to the general population. In the 1980s, a great deal of research implicated physical and

sexual abuse of children by parents as a significant factor in increasing the risk of psychological disturbance in adolescents, including suicide risk (Lester, 1992). These experiences are especially common in adolescents who run away from home and who are in shelters for the homeless.

From a clinical perspective, Bruce's family exhibited most of the preceding characteristics. Bruce's mother did not sufficiently differentiate her role from her sons. She herself relied on Bruce for her support. The family was inflexible. Not only Bruce, but also his brothers were secretive and hostile; his brothers also had been in trouble with the police. Bruce lacked communication skills. In his therapy sessions he often would communicate little. He would state, "It's your job; you talk." If questioned he would say, "Fuck you," stating he was there because his mother made him. With an adolescent so violent, one wonders how his mother managed to "make him" attend treatment. Was the force of the relationship that compelling? There was a very close attachment, despite Bruce's constant verbal attacks on her. There was a deep ambivalence, which in time became even more severe, as Bruce began deliberately to provoke his mother into open conflict.

Clearly, Bruce's family was dysfunctional. His mother saw her previous marriage as abusive, yet the divorce was traumatic as well. Bruce rarely saw his father after the divorce, stating "He's just my father; he doesn't live with us." He had little respect for and refused to listen to his father, who may have been an alcoholic. His brothers were heavy users of drugs and alcohol.

Bruce felt he had little control over his life and environment. He was depressed but expressed only anger, and his mother could not cope with his turmoil. The family became more dysfunctional. The exacerbation of problems in school only added to the disorganization.

AN IDIOGRAPHIC CONCLUSION

How suicidal was Bruce? At first there was a low suicide risk. This risk increased, as reflected in increased drug and alcohol use, anger and aggressiveness, nihilistic and pessimistic thought patterns, and self-destructive behavior. However, Bruce's level of lethality was constantly in flux. Sometimes it was low. Sometimes it was low-moderate.

It was never high while he was in treatment. Adolescent patients, in general, do not fit easily into our models, even into the concepts of lethality and perturbation. Overall, however, Bruce was at increased risk of suicide as treatment continued.

One night Bruce was arrested. He had been drinking and was charged with breaking and entering. Bruce was placed in a detention center where, six hours later, he attempted to hang himself. Upon inquiry, fellow inmates said they had warned the guards. One inmate said, "He was in the cell crying. He said 'Fuck—I'll kill myself.'" Bruce had then been placed in an isolation room where he was monitored every 20 minutes. In his suicide attempt, Bruce used a bed sheet, tied it around his neck, sat on the floor and choked himself, a frequent method of suicide in jails and hospitals. A nurse had evaluated Bruce upon his arrival and saw no risk for suicide, adding that all young offenders are at risk. An internal inquiry subsequently had been undertaken, ruling that all procedures were properly followed. Yet anyone with an understanding of suicides in jails would have questioned the level of assessment and subsequent monitoring that had occurred (Bonner, 1992). In fact, there are a host of complex issues in the assessment and prediction of suicide in such facilities (Litman, 1992), and there are legal and liability issues as well (Bongar, 1991).

What was Bruce's suicide risk? How lethal was the act? Our clinical judgment would be that it was moderate-high immediately preceding his attempt. He did communicate being suicidal. His attempt was in a public place. Perhaps it was more lethal because of the lack of adequate procedures at the jail. Clearly the isolation room made the suicide risk more severe.

On both the available scales—the BSIS (Beck et al., 1979) and the LSARS (Smith et al., 1984)—identified as useful by the NIMH group (Lewinsohn et al., 1989), Bruce's behavior would score in the moderate-high range. Using the terminology from the tests, we learn the following.

On the BSIS (Beck et al., 1979), a mixed picture develops, of the sort that usually suggests moderate to high lethality (Beck, Beck, & Kovacs, 1975). Bruce was isolated; he timed the attempt immediately after a guard checked in to monitor him. Intervention was unlikely, except that the guard did not adhere to the 20-minute schedule; she arrived sooner. Bruce made no final acts in anticipation of death and no attempt to get help. There was little preparation and no note; there was equivocal communication. His attempt was made both to change the environment and to remove himself.

In part, the BSIS is based on a patient's own evaluation. Did he want to die? Or did he want to change the situation? How serious was the act? Bruce's self-report, although essential for completeness with the BSIS, was not available. Third-party reports would have placed him at high risk ("Fuck, I'll kill myself"). The act was characteristically impulsive. Bruce thought that he would die, according to reports; however, his conception of the effectiveness of the method was somewhat inaccurate, which is a point worth noting in evaluations (Beck, Beck, & Kovacs, 1975). Finally, he had made no previous attempt, suggesting a lower score on the evaluation (Beck et al., 1979).

On the LSARS (Smith et al., 1984), the lethality of Bruce's act would suggest an estimate concomitant with the BSIS. He would score a 7.0, suggesting death is the probable outcome unless there is "immediate" and "vigorous" medical attention. He made a communication, and the act was performed in public, albeit in an isolation cell. Were it not for the guard, his score may have been higher (i.e., 8 or 9). Did he think, for example, that the act was in private? Was it an unforseen circumstance that the guard arrived earlier? Impulsive people, like Bruce, may be rash in their choice of method. Obviously, Bruce's own self-report is needed to make a more sound evaluation.

Assessment and prediction of suicide are complex and not always successful, but can be approximated and may well be life-saving. In Bruce's case, although he had been at moderate risk before his attempt, it would have been difficult to predict when, where, and how he would try to end his own life. Given his status as a suicide attempter at continued risk for self-destructive behavior, however, Bruce now represented new challenges for assessment and prediction as he was placed in a hospital setting (Litman, 1992). He was listed in critical condition. During the process of medical recovery and beyond, Bruce would require renewed demands for careful assessment in order to attempt to predict the likelihood of recidivism and to allow for the possibility of preventing it.

ASSESSMENT OF SUICIDE RISK: A SUMMARY

We have tried to underscore in this chapter that suicide is a multidimensional malaise. The ideas presented here for understanding of suicide and, by implication, assessment and prediction of suicide risk are only a beginning. We wish to make clear that predicting suicide is complicated and difficult, as demonstrated by the case example presented here: Bruce's risk obviously fluctuated, he responded excessively to every event, and there was a lack of sound personal (ego) functioning. Nevertheless, his life-threatening suicide attempt was not anticipated well enough to prevent it. Clearly, then, suicide assessment and prediction must be ongoing in our treatment of suicidal adolescents.

We also wish to emphasize that it is likely that no one behavior, including a test score, will provide all of the information needed to assess and predict suicide. Each bit of information (such as a test score, an observation) will have to be placed in the context of the life of the individual. It is likely that a number of tests, interviews, and scales will be needed in each case to predict such a complex human behavior as suicide. There is no one phrenological "bump on the head" that will tell us whether an adolescent is suicidal or not, much less how suicidal that person is. Furthermore, all predictions ultimately depend on the skill of the clinician. In that sense, suicide prediction is a task like many others that a sound clinician faces—a problem of understanding a number of ongoing evaluations of the same adolescent, and drawing hypotheses and conclusions from that group of evaluations in order to make effective clinical interventions that may save a life.

REFERENCES

American Psychiatric Association (1994). *Diagnostic and statistical manual of mental disorders* (4th ed.) (DSM-IV). Washington, DC: American Psychiatric Association Press.

Anastasi, A. (1982). *Psychological testing* (5th ed.). New York: Macmillan.

Barraclough, B. (1986). The relation between mental illness, physical illness and suicide. In J. Morgan (Ed.), *Suicide: Helping those at risk* (pp. 61–65). London: King's College.

Beck, A., Beck, R., & Kovacs, M. (1975). Classification of suicidal behaviors: I. Quantifying intent and medical lethality. *American Journal of Psychiatry, 132,* 285–287.

Beck, A., Kovacs, M., & Weissman, A. (1979). Assessment of suicide ideation: The Scale for Suicide Ideation. *Journal of Consulting and Clinical Psychology, 47,* 343–352.

Beck, A. T., Resnik, H., & Lettieri, D. (1974). *The prediction of suicide.* Bowie, MD: Charles Press.

Beck, A., & Steer, R. (1987). *Manual for the revised Beck Depression Inventory.* San Antonio, TX: The Psychological Corporation.

Beck, A. T., Weissman, A., Lester, D., & Trexler, L. (1974). The measurement of pessimism. *Journal of Consulting and Clinical Psychology, 42,* 861–865.

Berman, A., & Jobes, D. (1991). *Adolescent suicide: Assessment and intervention.* Washington, DC: American Psychological Association Press.

Blos, P. (1979). *The adolescent passage.* New York: International Universities Press.

Bongar, B. (1991). *The suicidal patient.* Washington, DC: American Psychological Association Press.

Bonner, R. (1992). Isolation, seclusion, and psychosocial vulnerability as risk factors for suicide behind bars. In R. Maris, A. Berman, J. Maltsberger, & R. Yufit (Eds.), *Assessment and prediction of suicide* (pp. 398–419). New York: The Guilford Press.

Corder, B., & Haizlip, T. (1984). Environmental and personality similarities in case histories of suicide and self-poisoning in children under ten. *Suicide and Life-Threatening Behavior, 14,* 59–66.

Corder, B., Parker, P., & Corder, R. (1974). Parental history, family communication and interaction patterns in adolescent suicide. *Family Therapy, 3,* 285–290.

Eissler, R., Freud, A., Kris, M., & Salmit, A. (Eds.) (1977). *Psychoanalytic assessment: The diagnostic profile.* New Haven, CT: Yale University Press.

Erikson, E. (1963). *Childhood and society* (2nd ed.). New York: Norton.

Erikson, E. (1964). *Insight and responsibility.* New York: Norton.

Erikson, E. (1968). *Identity: Youth and crisis.* New York: Norton.

Esman, A. (Ed.) (1975). *The psychology of adolescence.* New York: International Universities Press.

Eyman, J., & Eyman, S. (1992). Personality assessment in suicide prediction. In R. Maris, A. Berman, J. Maltsberger, & R. Yufit (Eds.), *Assessment and prediction of suicide* (pp. 183–201). New York: The Guilford Press.

Farberow, N. (Ed.) (1980). *The many faces of suicide.* New York: McGraw-Hill.

Freud, A. (1965). *Normality and pathology in childhood.* New York: International Universities Press.

Fryer, J. (1986). AIDS and suicide. In J. Morgan (Ed.), *Suicide: Helping those at risk* (pp. 193–200). London: King's College.

Garrison, C., Lewinsohn, P., Marsteller, F., Langhinrichsen, J., & Lann, I. (1991). The assessment of suicidal behavior in adolescents. *Suicide and Life-Threatening Behavior, 21,* 217–230.

Hathaway, S. R., & McKinley, J. C. (1967). *The Minnesota Multiphasic Personality Inventory: Manual for administration and scoring.* New York: Psychological Corporation.

Holmes, T., & Rahe, R. (1967). The social readjustment scale. *Journal of Psychosomatic Research, 11,* 213–218.

Jastak, S., & Wilkinson, G. S. (1984). *The Wide Range Achievement Test— Revised: Administration manual.* Wilmington, DE: Jastak Associates.

Johnson, J. H., & McCutcheon, S. (1980). Assessing life stress in older children and adolescents. In I. Sarason & C. Spielberger (Eds.), *Stress and anxiety* (vol. 7, pp. 111–125). Washington, DC: Hemisphere.

Kaufman, A. (1979). *Intelligence testing with the WISC-R.* New York: John Wiley & Sons.

Kazdin, A., Rodgas, A., & Colbus, D. (1986). The Hopelessness Scale for Children. *Journal of Consulting and Clinical Psychology, 54,* 241–245.

Kovacs, M. (1985). The Children's Depression Inventory. *Psychopharmacology Bulletin, 21,* 995–998.

Kral, M. (1992, April). *A model for psychological assessment of risk.* Paper presented at the 25th Annual Meeting of the American Association of Suicidology, Chicago, IL.

Laufer, M. (1975). *Adolescent disturbances and breakdowns.* New York: Penguin.

Leenaars, A. (1988a). *Suicide notes.* New York: Human Sciences Press.

Leenaars, A. (1988b, October). Preventing youth suicide: Education is the key. *Dimensions in Health Service,* pp. 22–24.

Leenaars, A. (1992). Suicide notes, communication, and ideation. In R. Maris, A. Berman, J. Maltsberger, & R. Yufit (Eds.), *Assessment and prediction of suicide* (pp. 337–361). New York: The Guilford Press.

Leenaars, A., & Wenckstern, S. (1991). Suicide in the school-age child and adolescent. In A. Leenaars (Ed.), *Life-span perspectives of suicide* (pp. 95–107). New York: Plenum.

Lester, D. (1974). Demographic versus clinical prediction of suicidal behaviors. In A. Beck, H. Resnik, & D. Lettieri (Eds.), *The prediction of suicide* (pp. 71–84). Bowie, MD: Charles Press.

Lester, D. (1992). *Why people kill themselves* (3rd ed.). Springfield, IL: Charles C. Thomas.

Lewinsohn, P., Garrison, C., Langhinrichsen, J., & Marsteller, F. (1989). *The assessment of suicidal behavior in adolescents: A review of scales suitable for epidemiological clinical research.* Rockville, MD: National Institutes of Mental Health.

Litman, R. (1992). Predicting and preventing hospital and clinic suicides. In R. Maris, A. Berman, J. Maltsberger, & R. Yufit (Eds.), *Assessment and prediction of suicide* (pp. 448–466). New York: The Guilford Press.

Maltsberger, J. (1992). The psychodynamic formulation: An aid in assessing suicide risk. In R. Maris, A. Berman, J. Maltsberger, & R. Yufit (Eds.), *Assessment and prediction of suicide* (pp. 25–49). New York: The Guilford Press.

Maris, R. (1985). The adolescent suicide problem. *Suicide and Life-Threatening Behavior, 15,* 91–109.

Marzuk, P. (1989, April). *AIDS-related suicides.* Paper presented at the 22nd Annual Meeting of the American Association of Suicidology, San Diego, CA.

Murray, H. A. (1943). *Thematic Apperception Test.* Cambridge, MA: Harvard University Press.

Peck, M. (1985). Crisis intervention treatment with chronically and acutely suicidal adolescents. In M. Peck, N. Farberow, & R. Litman (Eds.), *Youth suicide* (pp. 112–122). New York: Springer Publishing Co.

Pfeffer, C. (1981a). Suicidal behavior of children: A review with implications for research and practice. *American Journal of Psychiatry, 138,* 154–160.

Pfeffer, C. (1981b). The family system of suicidal children. *American Journal of Psychotherapy, 34,* 330–341.

Pfeffer, C. (1986). *The suicidal child.* New York: The Guilford Press.

Reynolds, W. M. (1986). *The Reynolds Adolescent Depression Scale.* Odessa, FL: Psychological Assessment Resources.

Rorschach, H. (1942/1981). *Psychodiagnostics: A diagnostic test based on perception.* New York: Grune & Stratton.

Rourke, R., & Fisk, J. (1981). Socio-emotional disturbances of learning disabled children: The role of central processing deficits. *Bulletin of the Orthopsychiatry Society, 31,* 77–88.

Rourke, R., Young, G., & Leenaars, A. (1989). A childhood learning disability that predisposes those afflicted to adolescent and adult depression and suicide risk. *Journal of Learning Disabilities, 22,* 169–175.

Sarason, I., Johnson, J., & Siegel, J. (1978). Assessing the impact of life changes. *Journal of Consulting and Clinical Psychology, 46,* 932–939.

Seiden, R. (1984). The youthful suicide epidemic. *Public Affairs Report.* Los Angeles: Regents of the University of California.

Shneidman, E. (1973). Suicide. In *Encyclopedia Britannica,* 21st ed., vol. 14 (pp. 383–385). Chicago: William Benton.

Shneidman, E. (1985). *Definition of Suicide.* New York: John Wiley & Sons.

Smith, K., Conroy, M., & Ehler, P. (1984). Lethality of suicide attempt rating scale. *Suicide and Life-Threatening Behavior, 14,* 215–242.

Steer, R., & Beck, A. (1988). Use of the Beck Depression Inventory, Hopelessness Scale, Scale for Suicide Ideation, and Suicide Intent Scale with adolescents. *Advanced Adolescent Mental Health, 3,* 219–231.

Toolan, J. (1981). Depression and suicide in children: An overview. *American Journal of Psychotherapy, 35,* 311–322.

Wechsler, D. (1974). *Manual for the Wechsler Intelligence Scale for Children—Revised (WISC-R).* New York: Psychological Corporation.

4

Crisis Intervention with Suicidal Adolescents
A View from the Emergency Room

ROBERT CATENACCIO

Crisis intervention with suicidal adolescents lies at the intersection of three types of therapy, each of which alone might make the clinician uneasy: crisis intervention per se, work with suicidal patients, and work with aggressive, hostile, or withdrawn adolescents. Given the patients' often perilous stabs at mastering helplessness, the natural wish is to have these volatile young persons put safely away. We may feel tempted to choose another line of work entirely. Yet the therapeutic yield for the time spent can be great, and the patients are lining up at the registration window as we speak.

To be situated in an emergency room is some comfort, of course; crisis work with the most severely suicidal, psychotic, or conduct-disordered adolescents is best done when hospitalization can be offered at any time as a frank alternative. Other supports make the emergency room ideal for such work: a holding room, which defines a safe space while risks are being estimated; the presence of clerical, nursing, and security personnel; nearby medical services; and access to tranquilizing medication. Yet it is quite unusual for us to use either restraints or on-site medication, and excellent crisis intervention programs are being run out of clinics as well.

More important is the availability of colleagues, for discussion, supervision, anxiety containment, telephone assistance, and at times cotherapy. At Jacobi Hospital our child crisis team at present consists

The author would like to thank Audrey Walker, M.D., for assistance on the references and bibliography for this chapter.

of five clinicians, and the constant interchange among us multiplies each one's effective experience by five.

The involvement of even one colleague is an enormous help. The care of children is inherently a cooperative endeavor, whether the team consists of two parents, or various relatives and neighbors, or teachers and guidance counselors, or state case workers, or the cluster of friends, often struggling themselves, that our adolescent patients so ingeniously recruit into their service. A great deal of our work is conducted via the telephone; holding the other end of every telephone line is another member of our ad hoc treatment team, and all together we bear up the safety net of information, concern, and commitment.

APPROACH

Many clinicians have some experience in treating adolescents or suicidal patients, or in doing crisis intervention, but few in the combination of all three. Here the whole may be less daunting than the anticipated sum of the parts, since many of the strategies conducive to success in any one of these intersecting domains also serve well in the others.

For example, if we consider crisis intervention from the standpoint of therapist role or stance, in general one strives to be pragmatic, active, explicitly empathic, authoritative, and yet altogether modest about what can and cannot be controlled or accomplished—a tall order, needless to say. These are also useful approaches, of course, in dealing with suicidal patients, who need a lot of structure and direction. Adolescents, more than children or adults, generally find passive, neutral therapists to be not so much facilitating as withholding: They want signals to be clear, as long as they are not overbearing or moralistic.

In an emergency room, the interview, as in all brief therapies, is diagnostic and reparative at the same time. Ideally, every question the therapist asks should bear a message of support or challenge, just as every instruction, suggestion, or directive serves as a probe, to gauge by the patient's reaction the available mental resources and the progress of the working alliance. Thorough assessment of the working alliance, patient ego functioning, and the family provide the stable tripod upon which the more narrowly focused assessment of suicidal risk must rest.

ALLIANCE

The working alliance is central to all psychological therapies of whatever duration or approach, yet never more so than here (Brenner, 1979). In the past 20 years, many studies on suicide have been epidemiological (Brent, Perper, & Moritz, 1993; Shaffer, 1974; Shafii, Carrington, Whittinghill, & Derrick, 1985), attempting to define and weigh risk factors, with the result that clinical judgment is now informed by a recognition of probabilities. Nonetheless, in doubtful cases a careful estimate of the working alliance—its inception, growth through the first session, transferential distortions, and resilience under the pricks of deflating interpretations or the press of a plain account of the facts—can clinch the choice between outpatient crisis work and the hospital unit.

If the family is fundamentally sound, we are willing to send home even patients who have made attempts of high intent and lethality, with an explicit contract establishing: (1) a return appointment the next day; (2) an assurance that there is no current suicidal intent; (3) a common understanding of the central problem; (4) a preliminary treatment plan; and (5) a backup plan, including contact persons at home and in the emergency room with twenty-four-hour availability, should the patient feel overwhelmed and once more suicidal.

But first, needless to say, we have to be pretty sure with whom we are dealing; after all, this is a life-or-death handshake. In order to contract meaningfully, then, we must have a strong relationship and a firm alliance, based on the clear-eyed judgment of both parties and on mutual trust, built rapidly during the first encounter. The high level of activity and engagement is designed not only so that the therapist can get to know the patient, but so that the patient can get to know the therapist as well.

ASSESSMENT OF EGO FUNCTIONS

The assessment of ego functions is the subject of volumes unto itself (Bellak, 1973); however, a few words here may be useful. Taken together, a reliable history and a mental status examination provide a surprisingly good store of information on the patient's specific strengths and weaknesses.

Repeated school failures, for whatever apparent reason, may signal undetected learning disabilities, which a brief cognitive screening can begin to confirm (Silver, 1989). Likewise, attentional problems may show up as impulsivity by history and as a scattered, impatient way of answering open-ended questions in the interview.

Difficulties with frustration tolerance, which show up as outbursts or reactive moodiness by history, can be quite evident in how the patient deals with the delays and petty annoyances of the evaluation procedure itself. The dark edge of paranoia may show up anywhere.

Following are some general guidelines for evaluation: Form some estimate of general intelligence, including both conceptual thought and problem solving ability. Do not be put off by the obvious inadequacy of the estimate, nor by niceties of fairness or correctness, but make the best guess you can. If you are assertive and fortunate, often you can locate school records and records of prior assessments and testing, so the current crisis can be viewed against a backdrop of previously sampled performances.

Above all, try to get a clear reading of the operative moral structures (Kernberg, 1984): Is the patient guilt-ridden, or grandiose and unrestrained; defiant, provocative, or cruel; opportunistic, easily swayed, or calculating; furtive or bold; ashamed or proud of nefarious exploits; anxious or cool; sporadically caring or a committed tough customer? Here, as elsewhere, err on the side of caution; without poisoning your mind against the patient, assume the worst. This is remarkably difficult for most therapists, as we are by and large a gentle-spirited lot, or passive-aggressive at worst, and tend to lack empathy for practitioners of an ethic we disapprove of. We have observed three common errors of judgment based on the clinician's understandable reluctance to empathize with antisocial behavior. Two tempting errors are to condemn the behavior and the patient together (the "hard-nosed" approach) or, alternatively, to redefine antisocial pathology as "masked depression," in order to preserve positive regard (the "bleeding heart" approach).

A third temptation in the assessment of moral pathology, rarer but more pernicious, falls to those therapists who themselves have significant antisocial trends, often masked by a crusading overidentification with the patient. In the first case, the clinician may fail through an unwillingness to work through initial resistances to treatment; in the second case, through a lack of limiting and structuring interventions; and in the third, through a proneness to paranoid collusions. Yet correct diagnosis here is essential, since, along with depressed and psychotic patients, it is the impulsive, antisocial, and substance-abusing patients, typically facing a disciplinary crisis, who are at greatest risk of actual completed suicide (Shaffer, 1974). The best guard against all such errors consists in the routine involvement of more than one clinician at some point in every case.

The heightened need to communicate and to involve others in crisis work increases the importance of the mental status examination. It should not be thought of as a set of questions, but rather as an organizational structure in the mind of the clinician, a format for reporting observations so that they may be shared easily and effectively (MacKinnon & Yudovsky, 1986). A good mental status exam is vivid and brief, uses frequent quotations and descriptions to support inferences, and clearly highlights what is essential. It ends with a diagnosis and a formulation, tying together key elements of the presentation and stating in one plain English sentence the heart of the matter. The formulation points the way directly to the treatment plan.

SUICIDALITY

Suicidality is itself a complex and heterogeneous set of attitudes and dispositions, as our case examples will bring out. When there has been a focal idea, threat, or act, I generally find myself making repeated passes at it, swooping back around to it at hinge points in the interview. Deal with the suicidal thoughts or acts at the start, for example, to establish the seriousness and the principal purpose of the patient's visit. Be concrete, specific, factual, but not exhaustive, and let the patient know that you will come back to the topic later on.

Return to it when you have an understanding of how stressors came together and brought the adolescent to such a choice, when you can plausibly say "Oh, now I see why you must have thought that killing yourself was a good idea." With this sort of empathic phrasing you show that the contemplation of suicide is not hopelessly bizarre or alien to human nature, and that you are not horrified or disgusted by it, though it is genuinely frightening.

In other words, you can spell out the adaptive function of both ideation and attempt, perhaps for the first time. As with all other symptoms, a degree of acceptance of the suicidal tendency encourages the patient to put aside rigid distancing defenses, such as denial, minimization, or isolation of affect, and to join with you in a sobering return visit to the scene of the trauma.

Often the actual attempt was undertaken in an altered state of consciousness, chemically induced or otherwise dissociated, and so may be largely unavailable to the patient's volitional memory. By appropriate pacing, silences, rhythms, and repetitions, the clinician may induce in the patient a state of concentration akin to a light trance, in which the details of the attempt, then the fantasies and the affects may return to full consciousness. Leave an ear tuned to the music of speech.

For the clinician who does not deal with large numbers of suicidal adolescents, it is difficult to remain calm. It may be helpful to recall that many studies have shown suicidal thinking to be extremely common in random samples of adolescents (Harkavy Friedman, Asnis, Boeck, & DiFiore, 1987; Rutter, Tizard, & Whitmore, 1981; Zimmerman & Morledge, 1992), yet completed suicide is a relatively rare occurrence. But faced with the individual patient, we cannot afford to be either alarmist or unconcerned, and neither pure statistics nor intuition serves as an adequate guide. Rather, further exploration is then called for to establish real risk.

Return for another pass at the suicidal thoughts or actions when you have a sense of the patient's emotional makeup, when you have heard how aggressive and depressive trends pressed forward at other key times in the patient's life: "So when you get to that particular state of mind, I see, you usually take it out on yourself." Externalizing defenses—that is, blaming others for everything—have generally already proven insufficient by this point, so when a characteristic thought or behavior pattern snaps into focus and is recognized as one's own, it can be a powerful experience: Senseless pain suddenly makes sense! Here we are speaking no longer just of assessment, of course, but of therapy.

The cognitive distortions that accompany and maintain depression have been fairly well studied (Beck, Rush, Shaw, & Emery, 1978); essentially, they are exaggerations. Beyond this, in the more disturbed patients, there may even be a tenacious commitment to self-denigration and self-abuse, based on a dual image of the self as, on the one hand, miserable and unworthy, and, on the other, cruel, masterful, and domineering. Generally, this matched pair of carefully scripted roles derives from actual experiences of ridicule and abuse (Herman, Perry, & van der Kolk, 1989; van der Kolk, Perry, & Herman, 1991);

internalized in this way, such repeated traumas are at least brought under the partial control of the individual. In the histories of suicidal adolescents, we almost always find a long, slow development of chronic disappointment and learned helplessness (Seligman, 1975) predating the growth spurt of hopelessness around the current crisis.

MEDICATION

This is not the place for a full presentation of pharmacologic options and rationales, but we cannot altogether omit so important a set of interventions from a general discussion of treatment. Briefly, medication is tailored both to the underlying diagnosis and to the target symptoms. (See also Chapter 12.)

Productive psychoses and paranoia usually require antipsychotic medication; if we are dealing with acute reactions, sometimes low doses produce rapid and gratifying results (Green, 1991). On occasion, if the patient has had a recent medical exam, and prompt psychiatric follow-up care is in place, we are willing to begin antidepressant medications, especially the selective serotonin reuptake inhibitors because of their relative safety and rapid action.

Some conduct disorders are built on a base of undiagnosed attention deficit hyperactivity disorder (August, Stewart, & Holmes, 1983); in such cases, psychostimulants can be very helpful, in conjunction with the appropriate educational and disciplinary structures. Likewise, we have found that beta blockers can be adjunctive to cognitive-behavioral and environmental approaches in helping explosive and aggressive adolescents to gain control of their anger, which they often experience as a terrifying and alien force within them (Green, 1991). Mood stabilizers, which could be quite effective for some of the emotionally labile and disruptive children we see, unfortunately require closer blood-level monitoring than we can manage currently. In no case is the medicine the whole treatment, but it sometimes has proven to be the key to the first door, allowing further treatment to proceed.

FAMILIES

For the troubled adolescent at risk, the family represents the external complement to the internal ego structures we have been discussing. In tandem, family and mental structures provide the dependability, containment, values, and controls that allow outpatient therapy to proceed, that give us the confidence to make treatment contracts and follow-up appointments, or that direct us, by their lack, to choose instead the safety of the inpatient unit (Gold, 1988).

People build up a vision of themselves slowly, partly by assessing how they truly do behave and partly through identifications with others. During adolescence, with the practicing of new roles and the relinquishing of old ones, strains appear in the developing coalition of the self; the changes in real and fantasy relationships then have their most direct impact. Many times a suicidal crisis is triggered by a rupture in a relationship, which represents not only the loss of a loved one, but also the loss or death of a part of oneself (Bowlby, 1961; Crook & Raskin, 1975; Zimmerman, 1993). Therefore, meetings designed to clarify and, if possible, repair real relationships can have an astonishing impact. At the start there may be a general reluctance even to get into the same room together, based on anger, mistrust, and the fear that only more conflict will result. Here the therapist must gain the trust of all parties through individual meetings before attempting anything more ambitious, as an enzyme bonds separately with the different proteins, then allows them to couple upon itself and move off together.

Many of the children and adolescents we see simply have no families; they are the victims of extreme social breakdown, and they have used up whatever few options life offered. The exhausted foster parent, or the group home, or the police, deposit these sad children on our officially responsible laps. While assessing them, we care for them, for an hour or a day, until the social service agency or the inpatient unit takes over. But in such all-too-frequent cases we are not practicing crisis intervention, for these children need far more; they need a home, naturally, and beyond that, a family life.

I am often asked if we see many crack-using teenagers. We see hardly any, in fact; I suppose they take a different path. What we do see are the children of chemically dependent parents, or of fathers who are shot dead or locked away in prison, and of mothers who died of AIDS. When a grandmother or an aunt is available to work with, as is often the case, we are on fairly solid ground. When the devastation is complete, and the patient is thrown on the mercy of the state, our function changes, and we become short-term consultants and case workers.

CASE EXAMPLES

The following are examples from our work in the emergency room at a major medical center in a large urban location.

Case 1—Message in a Bottle

Marilyn, age 13, swallowed six aspirins out of a nearly full bottle and then promptly told friends at school. She was a serious and successful girl with many friends, showing clear signs of a stable early upbringing. However, two years ago her father, a truck driver, began dealing and using cocaine, and Marilyn witnessed many severe arguments and fights between her parents, including one in which they stabbed each other. Twice her mother had left the home and stayed with her own parents, once taking Marilyn and her older brother along, and once leaving them behind so that they could continue at their old schools; each time she returned. In the past weeks, the father had run afoul of gangsters and was living under the constant threat of death.

Discussion. This case was unusual for us, because the strictly psychological side of the girl's problem cleared up so rapidly as she told her story. Essentially, all I had to do was listen and understand; her father's drug abuse was the grain of sand around which the symptom had been formed. Her act, though expressive of great sadness, anger, and frustration, was almost purely of the "message" variety; once the message was heard and responded to, the girl showed a calm determination to remedy the real situation. A deeper interpretation, which I briefly tried, that she was trying magically to substitute her death for her father's, did not apply. As she said bluntly, "He got himself into this; he's got to get himself out." Her goal was to strengthen her mother's resolve and to get our practical help in planning their exit from the home. She also accepted a referral for outpatient therapy.

Case 2—Caught Again!

Felicity, also 13, was brought in by her mother because she had tried to jump out of her fourth-floor window the previous night, an impulsive act of high lethality but only moderate intent, since her mother and 14-year-old sister were in the room at the time. That day they had come home earlier than expected, to discover Felicity in the house with a 20-year-old delinquent boy, instead of at school, and mother's exasperated recriminations had led to the suicidal act.

Two weeks before, her mother had caught her at home with two other friends, a boy and a girl age 17, all truant from school, but Felicity hurried to chain-lock the door so her friends could escape through the window while her mother raged impotently. The landlord of the housing complex recently had written them a letter threatening to evict the family for repeatedly allowing these neighborhood nuisances into the elevators and corridors. Both of the young men were former boyfriends of the 14-year-old sister, but she, as usual, remained apparently uninfected by their miasma of mischief, and continued along the high road, an honor student and the very soul of good sense.

The mother and sisters were close, and these desperate clashes around Felicity's misbehaviors, defiance, and deceit were recent events, dating from their move six months before; then they had left their old neighborhood, full of friends, and also, living across the street, the girls' father. Even though her own parents lived nearby, the mother, who worked and commuted long hours, felt painfully isolated, a divorced immigrant Italian woman in a close-knit Asian community. Her daughters identified with their father's Latino heritage. But Felicity's chronic sadness, low self-esteem, and even suicidal ideation antedated the behavior problems by many years; they had begun at least as early as her sister had started her intense and accelerated studies, and six-year-old Felicity would sit alone and idle with an aged grandmother, while her mother and sister toiled up the ladder of success.

Discussion. This is a less striking story, perhaps, than the previous one, but a tougher one to resolve. Although the presenting symptoms were of fairly recent onset and not unusual in adolescence, there was a chronic history of hurt and feelings of inferiority. Unlike the previous case, right and wrong were not so clear; if anything, the patient was "wrong" in that she was developing a conduct disorder. Her goal for the therapy was to be allowed to meet with her boyfriend. Her mother wanted to work it out somehow, but lacked confidence in her ability to set limits without starting fights. Here it seemed at first that dyadic therapy was the way to go, helping the mother and daughter to communicate clearly, negotiate, problem-solve, compromise.

For example, we took the patient's wild wish and attempted to domesticate it: Couldn't the mothers of the star-crossed lovers get to know each other as well? They did manage to speak on the telephone, but no face-to-face encounter ever took place, although they lived all of 50 yards apart. We next involved the sister, a person of considerable symbolic importance in the family, who had miraculously managed to remain on friendly terms with everyone concerned. Fortunately, she was a stable and good-hearted girl.

But to our surprise, Felicity and her mother were still not willing to give life together a fresh try, even after a second family session. The father, his new family, and the old neighborhood turned out to be more central than we had thought, and Felicity was happier and more responsible when we arranged for her to move in with them and assume the role of the eldest sister in that household. I felt as if I had tried key after key to open a locked door, never noticing the second door standing open beside it. In retrospect, the interventions seem too controlling, and too clever by half; fortunately, this girl was patient enough to hold out for what she really needed.

Case 3—Last Call

We met Samantha, a pretty and somewhat bedraggled girl of 15, on the morning after a bender. Following another pointless argument with her mother about whether she could go out after dinner, she headed across the street, met up with some drinking buddies, and began to consume copious quantities of malt liquor. Both her younger brother and her best friend tried to stop her, but she told them to go get lost. Eventually she made it back home, staggered up the stairs, and passed out on the floor of her room. Her mother could not rouse her and had her brought by ambulance to the pediatric emergency room.

Samantha had been an honor student until the end of eighth grade, but the next year the public high school loomed up vast and formless, and Samantha began to cut classes to hang out with a few like-minded peers. By year's end, she was failing and was forced to repeat the year; consequently, she asked her parents to put her back into the parochial school system. But now she found she couldn't stand all the rules and the discipline either at school or at home, and she became both openly rebellious and deeply discouraged.

She began drinking, usually with a group of neighborhood cronies, and then began taking small secret overdoses of this and that, half hoping she'd be found out, half hoping they would do her in. Her mood, sleep, appetite, and concentration were all sinking for months, and she felt only an aching hatred for her parents. In fact, toward her father, who had lately tried several times to discipline her, harshly and in anger, and who had been until a year ago her best friend, she now felt a murderous rage.

Discussion. What made this case particularly problematic, of course, was the coincidence of the depression and the drinking. We could get lost trying to figure out which was primary, in time or importance. Instead, we simply announced that both are problems and asked to hear about the depression first; the patient wanted first of all to be understood and only then, perhaps, assisted.

We began by treating this apparently trivial episode as a serious suicide attempt, by making it bear the weight of all prior attempts as well. The ingestions were solitary, inarticulate rituals of mourning for the girl's lost excellence in school, for the old love between her and her father, and for the manageable world of childhood, irrecoverably lost.

A process of spoken sorrowing then began between the patient and the clinician; it continued with the parents present, and subsequently at home afterward. This was possible in our work because we have affiliated clinicians who can make home visits. Specific activities were assigned for the father and daughter together, to provide not only real pleasure but also mild, realistic disappointment, in place of a bitterly cherished nostalgia. Put differently, an adolescent should feel that she is outgrowing her parents, not that she has been jilted by them.

Psychoeducation about depression, antidepressants, and then the effects of alcohol followed. Finally, the now-undeniable advisability of a program for chemical dependency was brought in, when other elements of the treatment, and therefore the basic trust of the treatment alliance, were already in place.

Case 4—Knocking on Heaven's Door

Tim, a tall, thin, scholarly looking boy of 15, was brought to the emergency room after an overdose. That morning he had been late getting going, and his mother was already in the shower. He pounded on the bathroom door. If he wanted to use the bathroom, she shouted out to him, he could go right ahead and come in, but she wasn't going to rush out after she'd been yelling at him to get up for an hour. Now, obviously a 15-year-old boy could not enter his mother's shower room, even though she had dared him to do so with her sarcastic permission. He called her every vile name under heaven, but still he had to wait upon her pleasure.

In the afternoon, upon returning from school, he discovered that he had no keys, for his mother had slipped them out of his pocket. She would not open the door. He could not go and stay with his grandmother, as he usually would, because he had recently had a major fight with her husband, when Tim had jumped in to protect her in a marital battle.

For a while he rang the bell and pounded on the door, fuming while his mother watched calmly from the window above. Then he ran to the corner, bought a pack of a common cold remedy, and, under his mother's gaze, choked down ten pills. She called an ambulance to have him taken to the hospital but refused to have him admitted to an inpatient service.

Tim had felt suicidal on and off for several months and depressed for several years. His relations with his mother had always been sour. He was hostile and oppositional, and she was exceedingly critical. Up to his teens, she had beaten him frequently, but she could not beat the stubbornness out. His four-year-old half brother was his mother's favorite, and there was no love lost between the boys, as Tim resentfully dragged him off to nursery school every day. Tim's ally was his maternal grandmother, who unfailingly supported him in his battles with his mother. His father lived in another country with a new family, and Tim's yearly visits left him feeling more cast off than ever. He was a pale, driven, perfectionistic student, who had taken a summer internship to become a research scientist, but he had no other interests and was largely isolated from his peers.

By the morning after he had taken the pills, when we spoke with him, Tim no longer intended to kill himself; still, he was far from hopeful about his long-term prospects. "I think it will all be over soon," he said.

Discussion. Tim and his mother had nothing but chilly anger to offer each other, and between mother and grandmother things were worse. For the follow-up appointment with Tim, the therapist was delayed, held an abbreviated session, and rescheduled for the next day; but Tim, perhaps put off by the perceived insult and readily lapsing into his customary hopelessness and passivity, failed to show up. On the telephone, he denied any current suicidal intent and showed no interest in returning to see us. Months later he was seen on the street, grimly hauling his little brother along to school.

A year later Tim made a second attempt under nearly identical circumstances. Can we then say, with the wisdom of hindsight, that we should have hospitalized him the first time, over his protests and his mother's—a course we almost never follow? Yet this second time he quickly allied with a therapist who saw him at home and who frankly validated his sense of his mother's almost homicidal hostility. Tim made the often difficult transition to long-term therapy at our clinic and appears to be doing well as he awaits his departure for college.

GENERAL THERAPEUTIC CONSIDERATIONS

Broken homes and multiple placements; repeated physical and sexual abuse; neglect, harsh and erratic discipline, and witnessed violence; learning disabilities, attention deficits, and school failures; extreme poverty across generations, with cultural displacement, deprivation, and disintegration; mental and physical illness in their caregivers; alcohol, drugs, and despair—this is a short list of the routine elements in the childhoods of the young people who come to an inner-city psychiatric emergency room. The sheer number and severity of life disruptions, beginning early on and continuing into adolescence, distinguish our suicidal adolescents from the merely depressed (de Wilde, Kienhorst, Diekstra, & Wolters, 1992).

How can our eyes pick out the defined edges of the current crisis against such a background? And how can we call hopelessness about oneself, the world, or the future a cognitive distortion when such have been the givens of experience? Yet remarkably, wonderfully, the vital energy of youth still seeks an outlet, an object, a life course. Often it is the very intensity of these teenagers' investment in the world that brings them to grief; a missed telephone call, a failed test, a scolding, a forgotten birthday, a jealous doubt, can snatch from them that promised salvation that had at last seemed within their grasp. Hope and hopelessness lie side by side, restlessly.

The Healer

It is easier, I think, than most dicta on troubled teens suggest to get on with them, to draw them out, at least in the heat of the crisis. In fact, the greatest danger for certain clinicians will come from their own charisma and availability, as models, saviors, mothers, and lovers for these hungry hearts. We must be careful always to promise less than we can deliver. Yet some interest and faith must be sparked between the clinician and the patient and between the clinician and the caregiver as well. While the tightly limited goals and hours of the therapy are being stated and restated, a second, implicit transaction is taking hold too— one of shamanic force: "I believe in you; you believe in me."

So, beginning with the most basic information gathering, the clinician balances quite consciously between denial and despair. The operative equation we are promoting is "Hope Means Work" and vice versa. Destructive behaviors must be identified and labeled, confronted with their derivation, result, meanings, and function, and then systematically replaced with preferable alternatives. This sort of work is no doubt already familiar to most clinicians under a variety of labels.

All potential allies should be pressed into service. We have found that school guidance counselors and homeroom teachers generally respect our presumed expertise and are delighted to receive both explanations and advice over the telephone. Especially for teenagers, their friends, boyfriends, and girlfriends can be quite as essential as blood relations. In dyadic or family sessions, recognition of interactional patterns and emotional states should be taught frankly, along with a few key rules and skills of effective communication; for example, no insults, stay on one topic at a time, focus on specifics, flexible brainstorming to solve problems cooperatively, when and how to stop a discussion that is heading for trouble. We do not hesitate to coin labels for common interchanges, to write down behavioral prescriptions or assignments. The session becomes a seminar.

Talking Tactics

At times, however, we meet not only with ignorance but with vigorous disagreement. The family's own experience may appear to argue against us, since the skills needed by both parents and offspring during the teen years differ sharply in many particulars from what worked before. In addition, resistance to taking advice may be heightened by a perceived incompatibility of cultures, by the mutual "foreignness" of client and clinician.

The role of culture in psychiatry is, I think, enormously underrated and is much too large and important a topic even to introduce here (McGoldrick, 1986). Suffice it to say that in short-term family-oriented work, at least, we play a losing game if we debate values and goals. Talk tactics. Most patients and parents will readily concede that theirs aren't working. The only convincing way to teach these skills is to demonstrate their effectiveness on the spot, by using them in the work and pointing out when you do so. Lay all your cards on the table.

For example, if you are trying to keep a mother and teenage daughter on topic when they are negotiating a curfew, and you fail a few times, shift your focus from the curfew to the communication skill they need to learn. Define the project, and give an assignment. Like a good teacher—or, for that matter, insurance broker—show what you have to offer, and invite skepticism.

A clinician may ask the same question of patient or parent as he might ask of a colleague, after hearing an exhaustively detailed and overwhelming case presentation: "So, what do you think is really going on here?" A wealth of hard-earned insight and good common sense may have been held in reserve. That and related questions such as "What were you trying to accomplish?" "What if you had said the opposite?" and so forth establish a framework of expectations in which patient and family are explicitly assumed to be active, creative, and adaptive at all times, as much in their symptomatic behaviors as in their collaboration with the clinician. Any move that unsettles long-held assumptions of determinism and doom is to the good.

In the same collaborative spirit, the clinician could ask "When you decided to come here, in what way did you hope we might be helpful?"; or, "Where would you like to go with this now?"; or, "What recommendations would you suggest I make?"

A leavening of humor from time to time can cast matters in a new perspective, if the manner is gentle; in no way does it diminish the weight of our limited but genuine expertise. On the contrary, the occasional authoritative statement will stand out sharply against a background of honest and well-deserved humility.

No notion, however far-fetched, should be discarded without a thorough accounting of pros and cons, with the goal of making up a full menu of courses for the consumer to choose from. This strategy conveys respect, teaches one good way of resolving an impasse, and prepares for the full resumption of responsibility by the family at the end of the brief intervention. It also cuts the therapist down to human size from the start, short-circuiting resistances based on devaluing the work that we do.

Interpreting

Dissociative defenses, denial, and splitting must be interpreted constantly, or they will sink the therapy; depressive exaggerations cannot be allowed to stand as an adequate picture of reality either. Yet direct confrontation, unless thoroughly prepared, will generally raise hackles and only call up more resistance. Ideally, you should point out these mental maneuvers to the patient a few measures after they occur, in a moment of calm, when the full capacity of observation is available. As a second choice, since calm is so hard to come by, interpret the denial during the despair, and vice versa.

For example, if a teenager is claiming that the imminent death of his mother from AIDS is "no problem," we might say, "It certainly makes sense to me to feel that way. If it were my mother, and there was nothing anybody could do to help, I'd try to think about it as little as possible. What would be the use of feeling horrible all the time? Then I'd always be suicidal." Now we can explore the most painful emotions safely, at one remove. That is, when the patient's defenses are up, providing a measure of protection against disorganizing affect, ally with him or her, and then talk about the affect.

Likewise, to challenge defenses of denial and action, choose a moment when the patient is expressing despair instead. Presented with a child's explicit hopelessness about the situation at home and at school, we must first empathize with the distress; for example: "It must be hard just to get through the day with all that going on!" Along with the patient, we emphatically tally up all the griefs and wrongs, and validate the perception of real external difficulties both acute and chronic (and, by brief asides, we may here reduce an exaggeration or two, dryly, in passing). But if we are thinking ahead, this is also the right time to prepare for the upcoming and inevitable switch to denial: "I guess most of the time you try your best to put these problems out of your mind altogether, if you can manage—pretend they're not real, or no big deal." Then bring in the prime example: "Like when you get drunk" or "like when you said before you didn't need any help, from me or anybody." A problem behavior is easier to acknowledge when it is seen as plausibly motivated, as a defense; and a characteristic defensive operation is thereby acknowledged as well.

From such a position of interest and respect for the patient's adaptive creativity, a clinician can thoroughly explore the when, the how, and the why of even the most unproductive and ill-favored mental and behavioral strategies, from minimizing to drinking, drug-taking, and compulsive thrill-seeking. Even suicide attempts and gratuitous violence must be approached with an understanding of their place in the patient's emotional economy. What seem to be stark and evident dangers can be measured properly only by a survey and a summation of both their outer and their inner dimensions.

THEORY AND PRACTICE

Diagnosis, consequently, must be understood in its broadest sense and should include a weighing of the patterns, powers, and motives of all players. A biopsychosocial model of human functioning is sufficiently broad-based to serve as a theoretical foundation for such a diagnosis, whereas purely psychodynamic, psychophysiological, or systems perspectives tend to magnify phenomena within their preferred field of focus.

Specific interventions, however, must be fine-tuned; in the course of a single case, the clinician often will shift paradigms and perspectives, choosing one or another microscopic view temporarily, for precise targeting. In such shifting and perilous circumstances the clinician and the patient cannot be wedded to any one dogma, not even eclecticism; we can only strive for realistic understanding.

The forces at play are furious but finite. The crisis, like a storm, comes to an end. Then it may seem that, viewed from the perspective of these children's larger circumstances, the help we lend so briefly has accomplished very little, for we cannot provide them with the fundamentally good life they need and so desperately long for. Every so often, at the imperfect end of a case, discouragement steals over us too, as it does so frequently with our patients.

Modesty therefore becomes us. Yet what ultimately enables us to speak with a circumscribed authority as well is a recognition of the actual boundaries of the work. On one side lie clear indications for giving over responsibility to a state agency or to an inpatient hospital unit; on the other lies the patient's private power to end his or her life. (Here I am not speaking of rights, only of ability.) Between these bounds it is possible for the therapist to find sufficient calm to attend to the task at hand, perhaps even to enjoy it.

REFERENCES

August, G. J., Stewart, M. A., & Holmes, C. S. (1983). A four-year follow-up of hyperactive boys with or without conduct disorder. *British Journal of Psychiatry, 143,* 192–198.

Beck, A., Rush, A. J., Shaw, B. F., & Emery, G. (1978). *Cognitive therapy of depression: A treatment manual.* New York: The Guilford Press.

Bellak, L. (1973). *Ego functions in schizophrenics, neurotics, and normals.* New York: Wiley-Interscience.

Brenner, C. (1979). Working alliance, therapeutic alliance, and transference. *Journal of the American Psychoanalytic Association, 27*(Suppl.), 137–157.

Brent, D., Perper, J., & Moritz, G. (1993). Psychiatric risk factors for adolescent suicide: A case-controlled study. *Journal of the American Academy of Child and Adolescent Psychiatry, 32*(3), 521–529.

Bowlby, J. (1961). Childhood mourning and its implications for psychiatry. *American Journal of Psychiatry, 118,* 481–498.

Crook, T., & Raskin, A. (1975). Association of childhood parental loss with attempted suicide and depression. *Journal of Consulting and Clinical Psychology, 43,* 277.

de Wilde, E., Kienhorst, I., Diekstra, R., & Wolters, W. (1992). The relationship between adolescent suicidal behavior and life events in childhood and adolescence. *American Journal of Psychiatry, 149*(1), 45–51.

Green, W. (1991). Principles of psychopharmacotherapy and specific drug treatments. In M. Lewis (Ed.), *Child and adolescent psychiatry: A comprehensive textbook* (pp. 778–782). Baltimore, MD: Williams and Wilkins.

Gold, J. R. (1988). An integrative psychotherapeutic approach to psychological crises of children and families. *Journal of Integrative and Eclectic Psychotherapy, 7,* 135–149.

Harkavy Friedman, J. M., Asnis, G. M., Boeck, M., & DiFiore, J. (1987). Prevalence of specific suicidal behaviors in a high school population. *American Journal of Psychiatry, 144,* 1203–1206.

Herman, J. L., Perry, C., & van der Kolk, B. (1989). Childhood trauma in borderline personality disorder. *American Journal of Psychiatry, 146,* 490–495.

Kernberg, O. (1984). Clinical aspects of severe superego pathology. In O. Kernberg, *Severe personality disorders* (pp. 275–289). New York: Wiley-Interscience.

MacKinnon, R., & Yudovsky, S. (1986). *The psychiatric evaluation in clinical practice* (pp. 58–84). Philadelphia, PA: J. B. Lippincott.

McGoldrick, M. (Ed.) (1986). *Ethnicity and family therapy.* New York: The Guilford Press.

Rutter, M., Tizard, J., & Whitmore, K. (Eds.) (1981). *Education, health, and behavior* (2nd ed.). Huntington, NY: Krieger.

Seligman, M. E. P. (1975). *Helplessness: On depression, development, and death.* San Francisco, CA: Freeman.

Shaffer, D. (1974). Suicide in childhood and early adolescence. *Journal of Child Psychology and Psychiatry, 15,* 275–291.

Shafii, M., Carrigan, S., Whittinghill, J. R., & Derrick, A. (1985). Psychological autopsy of completed suicide in children and adolescents. *American Journal of Psychiatry, 142,* 1061–1064.

Silver, L. B. (1989). *Assessment of learning disabilities, preschool through adulthood.* Boston: Little Brown.

van der Kolk, B., Perry, C., & Herman, J. (1991). Childhood origins of self-destructive behavior. *American Journal of Psychiatry, 148,* 1665–1671.

Zimmerman, J. K. (1993, April). *Loss and disconnection in adolescent suicide: A cross-cultural and female developmental perspective.* Paper presented at the 26th Annual Meeting of the American Association of Suicidology, San Francisco, CA.

Zimmerman, J. K., & Morledge, J. (1992). *Prevalence of specific suicidal behaviors in a high school sample: A replication and extension.* Unpublished manuscript.

5

Immediately after the Suicide Attempt
Evaluation and Brief Therapy on a Medical Ward

EVERETT DULIT

This chapter describes a particular service at a particular place at a particular time doing a particular job. My goal here is not to make overall statements about the phenomenon of adolescent suicide or even about programs intended to work with that problem. My goal instead is to characterize as well as I can one particular program that has emerged in the hands of my colleagues and me and to convey some critical features of how that program works and what we think is good about it. There will inevitably be many matters I could have addressed that I will not. So be it. My goal is clarity about what we *do*, clarity about some *ideas* we have about what we do, and clarity about why we think it is at least one reasonable way of working, particularly in a setting like ours.

Our setting is an acute Adolescent Medicine Service (not a psychiatry service) in an inner-city general hospital closely affiliated with a high-quality academic medical center. The patient population from which we draw is primarily blue collar through poverty (social classes III through V [Hollingshead, 1975]). The initial admission to this medical service is typically for the medical consequences of a suicide attempt, with an occasional patient admitted for suicidal ideation only. But the behavioral, psychological, and family dimensions of the situation are an early focus and become central as the medical problem resolves.

The key workers with the patient become "the behavioral team," one half-time liaison psychiatrist and one full-time social worker.

Both interview and work with the patient; the social worker does most of the work with the family. The psychiatrist becomes actively involved where that seems especially indicated. Decisions are always made jointly, with disagreements resolved in discussion, sometimes with input from the unit director (a pediatrician, nationally known for work in adolescent medicine, with a special interest in behavioral issues) who functions then as part of "the behavioral team."

The Adolescent Medicine Service has 20 beds, a house staff of about six, and a nursing staff of about eight on duty during daytime hours and four at night. There is also an attending on the ward who is a member of the senior pediatrics faculty. At any given time, we have an average of one to three adolescents on the unit who are there in the aftermath of a suicide attempt. The average stay is three to seven days (longer for the occasional serious placement problem). Thus in the course of a year we see approximately 100 to 150 cases, with about 10 to 15 percent being repeat attempts, most of those previously seen by us.

We begin our work with our adolescent suicide attempters by concentrating on making an evaluation. Although there is an infinitude of questions and issues that one may find oneself confronting in any individual case, we tend to organize our thinking primarily around what we identify as the central question and issue confronting us: Is this a patient we're going to be able to send home safely, usually with a referral to outpatient therapy, or is this a patient for whom nothing less restrictive than placement in a secure psychiatric inpatient service for protective custody and a trial of treatment will be safe and appropriate? That critical "fork in the road" is the central organizer to our thinking during the evaluation. It is the key decision we will be making while the patient is with us. Simultaneously, while our patients are with us, we are looking for and trying for every opportunity we can find to do some brief therapy to try to make some progress on some key underlying issues and to leave them *thinking* something important about themselves, about the event and its background. We do so because we are operating in a situation where the great majority of our cases (about 80 to 90 percent) will be going home rather than to any inpatient treatment facility (where we could have been sure that they would get some treatment). Further, of those we send home and refer to outpatient therapy, consistent with data from other centers (Clarke, 1988; Rotheram, 1990; Trautman &

Rotheram, 1986; Zimmerman & Asnis, 1991; see also Chapter 6), only a very modest percent (5 to 10 percent) actually follows through on treatment despite our recommendations and referrals for follow-up psychotherapy. As a consequence, we work with the assumption that what we don't do in a trial of brief therapy while they are with us just won't get done at all, period.

EVALUATION

As we try to think our way through the evaluation issues in each individual case and through the brief therapy issues (i.e., on which features of the situation we should choose to focus and how to address them), our thinking tends to be organized around certain prototypical symptom constellations.

Type 1: Sudden Crisis State, Against a Background of No Substantial Prior or Current Psychopathology

A typical example would be the adolescent girl who has a rather well defined crisis, usually in her relationship with her mother (sometimes father or both parents), commonly around an issue involving boyfriend (curfew, suspicions or discoveries of sexual activity), often involving trust, rules and/or duties (e.g., aforementioned boyfriend issues, care of siblings). The method of suicide is most commonly pills in modest (3 to 5) to moderate (10 to 15) numbers, but occasionally much higher. The communication of intent is usually fairly straightforward—angrily locks self in bathroom and is heard taking pills, begins to feel sick and gets worried and tells—with minimal wish, effort, or effectiveness at concealment. The interview discloses no convincing evidence for substantial prior or current background of psychopathology.

Type 2: Current Episode Is Against a Background of Chronic Impairment of Ego Functioning in the Adolescent

This adolescent has made one or more previous suicide attempts and appears to function generally at a "borderline level" (i.e., we have some sense that Borderline Personality Disorder [American Psychiatric Association, 1994] is possibly a valid diagnosis). Our main initial working criteria for that diagnosis are a life of recurrent emotional storms and much serious mismanagement and ineffectiveness in handling the ordinary tasks of adolescence within school, peer group, and family.

Type 3: Mood State of Depression Seems Primary Causative Factor

This is an adolescent for whom there is nothing or relatively little in the story by way of precipitating factors, but who made the suicide attempt primarily because he or she was "feeling really down—life just didn't seem worth living." The emotional tone in these cases is most usually straightforward sadness and devitalization, with depletion of energy; by contrast, in Types 1 and 2, the dominant emotional tone is more usually active distress and anger.

DISPOSITION

Our thinking and initial direction for each of these types tends to be as follows.

Type 1

We assume these adolescents will go home and to outpatient therapy. They are seen most often in individual therapy, with only occasional sessions with parents, but sometimes are seen regularly with parents in an attempt to focus on the troubles in the relationship.

However, if this is a second or third attempt, we are very likely to insist on sending them to a psychiatric inpatient service, partially to communicate the seriousness of the behavior and/or to provide the opportunity for more extensive/intensive work.

Type 2

For Type 2 adolescents, we are much more likely to insist on a period of treatment in a secure psychiatric inpatient service, for more extensive evaluation and a serious trial of therapy in hospital. This is based on the assumption that chances of at least "engaging" a borderline adolescent and "borderlinogenic" family in therapy are a bit greater in hospital than out. Also we want to be using the insistence on hospitalization to be saying: "This is serious!"

Type 3

Our thinking in these cases is that the main causative pathway seems to be endogenous depressive factors rather than exogenous precipitating/causative factors. We are inclined here strongly toward recommendation of a trial of antidepressant medication, either in hospital or out (depending on safety and cooperativeness considerations).

ASSESSMENT

The clusters we have called Types 1, 2, and 3 occur frequently enough to make that typology useful as a first approach to thinking about evaluation in our setting, given the decisions we have to make and the dispositions we have available to us. Clearly, mixed cases and shades of gray appear all the time. However, the relatively simple typology just outlined covers the important facts and leads to what seem reasonable decisions, even in long retrospect, in an impressive number of cases.

As we conduct our initial interviews, we've found some questions to be particularly fruitful of useful answers:

To those who took pills we ask: "How many, roughly, did you take?" We think of ingestions of two to four pills as primarily a communication with minimal or modest intent to die, 10 to 15 pills as getting serious, and 20 to 40 as quite serious. Our general impression is that the "psychological magnitude" of the number of pills taken is a fairly good correlate of the seriousness of the intent to hurt oneself regardless of the particular drug taken, because generally our patients know very little about the relative toxicity of the drug they've taken. (Commonly they don't know its name, let alone its toxicity.) The larger numbers commonly represent serious intent to die, and virtually always they represent a measure of the severity of the feelings of distress experienced by the adolescent. The judgment of seriousness of intent is, to be sure, based only partially on number of pills taken. Such issues as expectable likelihood of discovery; words and feelings expressed before, during, and after the ingestion about intent to die; and other highly individualized factors also prominently influence this judgment. Nevertheless, we tend to think of number of pills as giving a handy and even quite reliable first approximation to seriousness.

Our next question to those who took pills is: "When you took those pills, did you think that that amount would be enough (or would *probably* be enough) to make you die?" If the patient says "yes," or was willing to take that chance, our next question is: "Well, clearly you've ended up alive after all. How do you feel about that? Glad you've ended up alive? Or sorry, and thinking maybe it would be better if in fact you *had* died?" The great majority of our patients say that they are glad they didn't die and make some statement like "It was a *stupid* thing to do!" Usually they say that with much feeling, sometimes undoubtedly for show, saying what they think they need to say to get out of the hospital—but more usually they seem to be speaking quite honestly. Only very rarely do we get a patient who says: "I'm sorry I didn't die. That would have been better." Such patients sometimes even add that they will "do it right the next time." It doesn't require experience to recognize that those patients are at very high risk. However, our experience has led us also to be quite alert for and to worry about the patient who shrugs, makes a face, and says: "I don't know." That response is not as dramatic as "I'm sorry I didn't die" but is far more common; undoubtedly, it also suggests high risk or at least higher-than-average risk.

If the patient says that she or he wasn't trying to be dead, then we ask quite seriously and persistently: "Then what *were* you trying for?" It is quite important to help the patient to realize that we're *not* trying to get them, as many tend to think, to criticize themselves as "having wanted to get attention" or anything like that. Adolescents tend to feel that we are trying to lead them into a speech saying: "I did a bad thing and I admit it now." They certainly do sometimes indeed have exactly that kind of an experience with parents, teachers, and others. That kind of speech would lead to a certain conventional kind of social and psychological closure, to a ritual of contrition. That, of course, is *not* our intent. It takes a little work, but usually one can manage to get the adolescent to see that we really are wondering: "If ending up dead wasn't on your mind, then what was?" We try to help them realize that there might well be a real answer. Some of the fairly clear and real answers we get from our patients are of the form: "I wanted to let them know how upset I was," or "I wanted to get them upset, and to realize . . ." or "I wanted to make them feel sorry." These answers identify those particular suicide attempts as a kind of expressive outburst or attempt at revenge, but not necessarily done with intent to die. In such cases, we always do make a point of emphasizing: "Even if you didn't really want to end up dead, you took a big chance on actually dying by taking pills. You don't know how many you could really take safely and not die; I'm a doctor and *I'm* not sure *I* would know for sure. And there are certainly safer ways of shocking people and getting them to sit up and take notice." We then go on to consider some of those other ways.

Commonly, after they state what they hoped the suicide attempt might accomplish—for example, catching the attention of parents—

our next question tends to be: "Did it work?" If the answer is yes, we tend to say "That's good," if it got them the attention, sympathy, and reconsiderations they were seeking. However, we also always emphasize the theme: "That also leaves me worrying that you might try the same thing again the next time you feel that you might want to achieve the same goal." That expressed concern leads naturally into a discussion about what to do instead any next time the impulse strikes again to use suicide as a means of communicating to and/or influencing others.

It's important also to note that often there does not exist a clear and real answer to our next question: "If it wasn't being dead that you were trying for, then what *were* you trying for?" Often the truth is served instead by some version of "I wasn't *thinking* anything" or perhaps yet more clearly: "I was just *so* upset. *That's* what I *was. Upset!* And *not* really thinking!" The frequency with which we get some version of that answer leads us to think it important to highlight here that the interviewer must be careful not to force or lead the patient into a statement implying more intentionality in the mind at the time of the attempt than captures what really happened. Often the adolescent's state of mind is more nearly captured by the notion that what was experienced was a storm of feelings combined with the idea: "I've just got to do something!" That conceptualization makes the event more like an act of reaction to and expression of those feelings rather than an act of intentionality. As part of that way of looking at the event, we resist interpretations that invoke alleged ideas of what the patient "was really thinking" (i.e., unconsciously). There is a strong tendency in psychological work to use the word "really" for something not visibly present but supposedly perceived by the professional observer "through" or "behind" the observable surface. Although such hypotheses are sometimes correct, we are skeptical of and resistant to easy access to that line of thought, and prefer to organize our own thinking more around what is directly perceived by the patient and ourselves. In our opinion, placing our focus on the surface of the patient's thoughts and feelings tends to pay off in material that we can use very directly in brief therapy. Thoughts and feelings directly perceived by patients are far more likely to be experienced by patients as part of "the truth in their lives," by contrast with material not directly perceived by them, and that tends to carry the therapy forward more rapidly.

BRIEF THERAPY APPROACHES

For us therapy begins with our initial contact with the patient. For example, it is commonplace in our first interview that a patient who has taken an overdose will say "I did a stupid thing" and "I'll *never* do it again." We are likely to respond: "I really am glad to hear you saying that, as compared to you saying the opposite. But—I *am* wondering—what makes you so *sure* of that?" Then, almost regardless of the response, we say: "You know, it really isn't so easy to be sure about what one is going to do in the future. For example, I'm sure you know as well as I do of people who really do want to do something like smoke less or eat less or anything like that. Such people often say to themselves and to others 'I'll never do it again,' and they really mean it when they say that, just like I'm betting you do also. But when it comes to actually smoking less or eating less, they find it hard to actually do. Often when the impulse to do the 'not-so-good' thing comes, they find it hard not to give in to that impulse. What makes you so sure you'll be able to resist, especially if it comes at a time when you're feeling again as upset as you were when you last did it, which happily you are not right now?" However the patient responds, with that line of thought one has moved directly into the beginning of a trial of brief therapy. If the patient has any capacity at all for thinking about thoughts and feelings, asking "How can you be so sure you won't?" usually leads you immediately onto very useful ground, as follows.

Sometimes the adolescent replies: "I would never want to end up *here* again! It was terrible. That *charcoal* that they make you swallow in the Emergency Room! Never again!" One problem for me, as listener to that statement, is the thought that I always have privately, in reaction: "Yes, but if you again become suicidal, you could avoid the charcoal and all the unpleasantness associated with being in the hospital by making your next attempt using a much more lethal method, for example by jumping off a roof." I don't say that, of course, but I'm not so reassured as the adolescent wants me to be.

Sometimes the adolescent says something like: "I just know. Maybe you don't believe me. But I know. I know I wouldn't." To which I usually reply: "Convince me." To which he or she usually asks, "How?" To which I usually answer: "Beats me. It's up to you. Go. And good luck." Typically, that leads to a conversation characterized by an interesting mix of relaxed humor with not-at-all relaxed tensions, by the communication of an honest willingness to be convinced side by side with a cheerfully conceded unwillingness to believe everything the adolescent says. That mix creates a tone for the interaction, honest and direct, that we experience as particularly favorable to facilitating brief therapy. It's a straightforward interchange, with real tensions, but with the professional evincing real friendliness and a real commitment to trying to be helpful. It accepts the truth that sensible people don't necessarily believe everything that other people tell them, particularly when there's a possible motive for purposeful deception and/or wishful self-deception by the speaker. It also assumes that both parties had best begin by simply acknowledging that fact and then get to work trying to find some way around that difficulty.

Developmental Issues and Therapeutic Responses

Two features of adolescent psychology that are centrally relevant in our brief therapy work with adolescent suicide attempts are a relative overvaluation of and reaction to emotionally "hot" current issues compared to relatively little valuation of the ability simply to survive "the slings and arrows of outrageous fortune"; and a "faulty" sense of the passage of time, one year feeling like a very long time and two years like an eternity.

Young people are highly likely to overvalue and overreact to emotionally charged issues in the here and now, which are likely to provoke the reaction: "I gotta do *something!*" In contrast, they are inclined to assign taking "the long view" a lesser importance, especially when the optimal response is not action but inaction, patience, and forbearance. Of course that tendency—overreaction to highly charged here-and-now issues and insufficient weight given to long-term implications—is not confined to young people. However, there appears to be a trend for that tendency to be greater in youth and significantly lesser in adulthood, as impulsiveness and the drive to action settle down somewhat and the capacity for considered reflection develops somewhat more fully. Compatible with that idea is the fact that we tend to say of adults for whom this does not much happen that they "haven't grown up" and "are still pretty adolescent in their ways."

A way of highlighting this issue and trying to make some headway with it has emerged for me in the course of working with suicidal adolescents. To me, it is important to find an effective way of saying to our patients: "That which has gotten you upset is very important, but not ending your life is infinitely more important!" It is easy, in the course of emphasizing the importance of the second issue, to appear (to the adolescent) to be playing down the importance of the first issue. That is especially problematic for those many adolescents who are so strongly in the grip of all-or-none, black-and-white thinking as to be virtually unable on their own to think in terms of shades of gray and relative weights of multiple considerations. For those to whom things are either "fantastic" or "it sucks," the shades of gray in life and all the middling measures are simply absent.

An approach that has emerged for me and that seems to do rather well as communication has been to say: "You know, if we were to take a scale, like a balance in which you weigh things, with one pan over here and the other over there [here I gesture with right hand as pan, and left hand as other pan], and if we put the problems that have you so upset into this right-hand pan, that would go way down." And when I say that, I drop the appropriate hand toward the floor, as if it is being weighed down with a quite substantial weight. Then I say: "But if I put into this other pan the importance to you ending your life, that completely flips the scale the other way!" I accompany that comment with a gesture of the "killing yourself" pan completely outweighing the "troubles" pan. That way of speaking and the movements that go with it work very well to communicate the idea: "As important as was the issue that was troubling you—and it *was* important—not killing yourself and staying alive is infinitely *more* important."

The critical question, of course, is whether this stance is convincing, whether it lasts in the mind, and whether it comes to mind the next time the adolescent faces a similar issue. My assertion would be that it does seem to communicate well, and communication certainly is the initial goal of a brief therapy. As to the degree to which it changes the patient's future, compared with what it might otherwise have been, that is difficult to be sure about, of course; there does seem real grounds for hope when we see, as we often do, that we stimulate real rethinking in the patient.

As for the second issue, which I called "faulty" time sense, I have in mind the tendency of young people to experience one year as a l-o-o-o-ng time, by dramatic contrast with what one year feels like in middle or especially later adulthood, when one year virtually "zips by." I put quotation marks around the word "faulty" because clearly the truth is more nearly served by the more even-handed perspective that the subjective sense of time is different earlier in life than later in life. For adolescents four years (the high school years) certainly seem like a whole era in life, while for their parents those same four years go by far more rapidly. Nevertheless, I do allow myself to use the word "faulty" to emphasize the degree to which adolescents' time sense can cause trouble. It can lead them to experience as "an eternity" a stretch of time (one year or two years) that they can and should be expected to "tough out." Because a year or two does feel like an eternity, some adolescents choose to kill themselves as a means of "opting out" of that anticipated "eternity" in a bad situation in the family or in the school. To be willing to throw away the entirety of the rest of one's life to escape a falsely anticipated "eternity" is what I am attempting to convey with my phrase "faulty sense of time."

An approach has emerged in our work that highlights the forgoing issue and tries to make some headway with it. At some point in our conversation with our adolescent patients, I say to them something like: "You know, if you do stay alive, you'll get to be 18 and 20 and 23 and 25 and 29 and 34 and 38 and 40 and 45, etc. . . ." (I purposely "draw it out" in my choice of words and in my tone of voice, which are calculated to create the feeling of a l-o-o-o-ng stretch of time unfolding in front of them.) "And that person who will be there in the world, who will be 35 or 40 or 45 and who will have your name and who you will become——that person will be you in some senses and will be quite different than you are now in some ways you can't even anticipate. And in an interesting kind of way, that person's life is in your hands! If you kill yourself now, that person is dead. And I can tell you, if you could somehow magically travel in time into the future and ask that person if she or he would want you to make a move now that would deprive her or him completely of any chance at life, I can tell you right now, that person would say: 'Don't do it!!'" Usually I stop right there, for maximum dramatic effect. However, if the adolescent seems to want to talk more about it, I may go on to say: "And I can even tell you something about *why* that person—you later on—would say that. Because there are pleasures to be had in life, pleasures you haven't begun to have and probably haven't even begun to know much about yet. But, boy, they are there to be had in life, and if you can just 'tough out' the bad stuff now, that future self of yours is going to have a chance to be in on some very good stuff. But if you end your life now, that person will be dead also and will never get to that good stuff."

My intent there is to "reframe" suicide so as to bring it closer to murder—of one's future self—based on my firm impression that most people (adolescents included) have much stronger internalized prohibitions against murder than against suicide. Suicide can feel to adolescents like something that concerns "only me" and so: "If I want to, who else am I hurting?" Of course one major answer to that question is family. However, feelings may be mixed about family and include some substantial wish to hurt. Therefore, I seek to introduce "future self" as an innocent bystander they would certainly hurt, whom they would indeed be murdering. It does leave them thinking. So also, more quietly, does the idea that there is life after adolescence and that just being able to "take it" can be a very praiseworthy thing.

Decision to Utilize Hospitalization as the Treatment Modality

There are two other features of our treatment of suicide attempters on our Adolescent Medicine Service. At time of admission and evaluation in the emergency room, our stance is: "When in doubt, admit." This is contrary to the working stance on most psychiatric services, which are understandably motivated to "protect" limited bed availability and to refer immediately to outpatient care any case seen in the emergency room where that seems at all feasible and responsible. Our intent is to communicate to adolescent and parents that "this is serious"; to give our behavioral team at least two to three days to evaluate and to try to make a potentially useful impact on family dynamics; and to provide a protected "time out" for all concerned, which almost always turns out to help. Thus we admit after every actual attempt, and sometimes for suicidal thinking and/or talk only, especially if new, especially if forceful.

When it happens that our recommendation for transfer to a psychiatric hospital is flatly refused by a parent, whom we had expected to be using as "petitioner" on the involuntary commitment form, we try if we possibly can, in good professional conscience, to tell that parent that "We really think you are making a mistake, but we will go along because we do not want to become the enemy and have you in a fight with us." We then add, "But if it looks to you over the next few days or weeks like maybe we were right and you also begin to feel really worried again—as we still are—don't be uncomfortable about calling us and saying that you are again more worried, and that maybe we should go ahead with the psychiatric hospitalization after all. You can be 100 percent sure that we will *not* be saying 'we told you so' or anything like that. We do want to help here, and it would not be good if you felt you couldn't call. So please do call us if you get worried again."

Our goal is to try to avoid becoming an adversary to the family if that is at all professionally defensible. In general, that seems to pay off in a better working relationship over the next few months or even years, as those families and adolescents often come to our attention again. Much less frequently, however, we do choose straightforwardly to become the adversary and to say to the family that we'll fight them in court and get the hospital administration to be the petitioner. So far, we've only done that about five times in a decade, and the family always eventually has conceded, without our actually having had to go to court to present our case. In such cases we've judged that the risks associated with not hospitalizing outweigh the disadvantages of creating an adversarial relation between ourselves and the family. Our prior experience in the courts leads us, almost universally, to expect support from judges for our petition when we assert: "This is a high-risk case, your Honor, and we strongly urge involuntary protective custody in hospital for a period of further evaluation and treatment. Discharge from hospital, even to outpatient treatment, is too likely to lead to death to be safe." No judge, in my experience, has ever overruled that.

SUMMARY

Because our adolescent patients are so poorly compliant with outpatient treatment as a general rule, our working hypothesis is that the only treatment our patients will get will come from us. As a consequence we concentrate on trying to accomplish what we can by way of brief therapy done in the three to seven days we have with these patients. Where turmoil and disconnectedness in the family appear to be a major contributing factor, we attempt to help the family to do better. Moreover, we always try to find a way to help the adolescent to live with what is likely not to get better in the family. We call it, pointedly, "survival techniques." We try to shape the brief therapy as a challenge to the patients and, it is hoped, as a memorable encounter. We tend to respond to their assurances that "it was a stupid thing" and "I'll *never* do it again" by saying that we're glad to hear them saying that, and we believe that they are really thinking it. However, we try to leave them realizing that sometimes such things are not as easy to carry off later as it feels now while they are still "in recoil." We try to leave them thinking about that, and we try to arm them with thoughts and plans about what to do then: "Call someone! Us, your best friend, someone in the family, any adult you like and trust, anyone who can help you fight off that impulse." We sometimes try to play the role of the "Benign Elder" by asking adolescent and parents: "Go now and be good to each other, because family is important, and family is for the purpose of helping people to live. To the outside world you may be no one special, but in the family you should all treat each other like someone special." Much less frequently we give advice that in some ways is the opposite. Where we think an adolescent is justifiably angry at a parent and is "turning the anger inward" (and where we feel that the anger will not go beyond words), we encourage the freedom to express that anger at someone in the family, including a parent, against whom an adolescent has legitimate grounds. Further, we try to ease the way for the adolescent by speaking ourselves with the parent about the "understandability" of the anger.

Where we think a key factor is a loss of a reasonable sense of proportion about the weight of the current difficulty versus the much greater weight of actually ending one's life, we use our metaphor of the scale and the balance pans. Where we think that a key factor may be the adolescent's foreshortened sense of time, we use our "if you stay alive you'll get to be 18 and 20 and 22 and 25 and etc." speech, trying to make real and even intense for the adolescent the sense that there is a long stretch of time ahead for living and for change and for adventure and for pleasure. We try to cap that by creating a concrete sense in the room of their "future self" who would want to live and not to be "murdered."

We also emphasize that the suicide attempt is not a strictly private matter but one that powerfully affects others: "Anyone who cares about you at all is tremendously shaken by the attempt, when happily you survive. And if you die, people who love you never fully recover, but live the rest of their lives hurting from having had that experience in their lives."

Finally, because research on suicide prevention is so very difficult, especially given the relative infrequency of the event, we certainly cannot pronounce with confidence about the effectiveness of our approach, compared to other approaches or to no effort at all. However, just as our patients often make a suicide attempt because they feel that they "have to do something!" about difficulties that confront them, so also do we, with a far more productive intent, feel that we "have to do something" that might help while we have the chance, even without research data confirming effectiveness. We even dare to think that what we do does help. Sometimes. And that's what we're trying for.

REFERENCES

American Psychiatric Association (1994). *Diagnostic and statistical manual of mental disorders* (4th ed.) (DSM-IV). Washington, DC: American Psychiatric Association Press.

Clarke, C. F. (1988). Deliberate self poisoning in adolescents. *Archives of Disorders of Childhood, 63,* 1479–1483.

Hollingshead, A. B. (1975). Two factor index of social status. New Haven, CT: Privately printed.

Rotheram, M. J. (1990, October). *The treatment of adolescents who have attempted suicide.* Institute presentation at the Annual Meeting of the American Academy of Child and Adolescent Psychiatry, Chicago, IL.

Trautman, P. D., & Rotheram, M. J. (1986, October). *Referral failure among adolescent suicide attempters.* Poster presented at the Annual Meeting of the American Academy of Child Psychiatry, Los Angeles, CA.

Zimmerman, J. K., & Asnis, G. M. (1991, August). *A multifamily intake group in a program for suicidal adolescents.* Paper presented at the 99th Annual Convention of the American Psychological Association, San Francisco, CA.

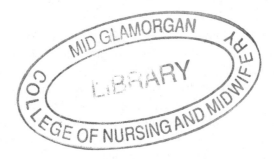

6

Enhancing Outpatient Treatment Compliance
A Multifamily Psychoeducational Intake Group

JAMES K. ZIMMERMAN,
GREGORY M. ASNIS, AND
BRUCE J. SCHWARTZ

Adolescent suicide is currently the third leading cause of death in 15- to 24-year-olds (National Center for Health Statistics, 1992). Therefore, the identification of effective ways of engaging and retaining at-risk adolescents in treatment is crucial. However, adolescents and their families often have been found to have a poor record of compliance and follow-through in treatment for a wide range of psychiatric and medical problems (Cavanaugh, 1990; Clarke, 1988; Joshi, Maisami, & Coyle, 1986; Kolko, Parrish, & Wilson, 1985; Nazarin, Mechaber, Charney, & Coulter, 1974; Vikander et al., 1986; Weighill, Hodge, & Peck, 1983), including referrals made consequent to suicide attempts (Clarke, 1988; Rotheram-Borus, 1990; Swedo, 1989; Trautman & Rotheram, 1986). Specifically, Rotheram-Borus (1990) reported that 20 percent of families of adolescent suicide attempters did not attend their first appointment for psychotherapy, and an additional 47 percent attended fewer than three appointments. In total, then, 67 percent of cases evidenced initial noncompliance or early dropout from treatment. In another study, Clarke (1988) found that 54 percent of adolescent suicide attempters were noncompliant or were early treatment dropouts when referred for psychotherapeutic follow-up after psychiatric hospitalization. Similarly, Swedo (1989) found that only 38 percent of adolescents psychiatrically hospitalized following a suicide

106

attempt followed through with outpatient psychotherapy despite having a discharge plan in place.

A number of reasons have been advanced to explain poor attendance at initial treatment appointments in a variety of medical and psychiatric settings. For example, variables such as low socioeconomic status (Alpert, 1964; Badgley & Furnal, 1961; Frankel & Hovell, 1978; Swenson & Pekarik, 1988), racial background (Adebonojo, 1973; Alpert, 1964; Badgley & Furnal, 1961; Frankel & Hovell, 1978; Swenson & Pekarik, 1988; Weighill et al., 1983), distance from clinic or unavailability of private transportation (Campbell, Staley, & Matas, 1991; Dubinsky, 1986; Swenson & Pekarik, 1988; Weighill et al., 1983), a lack of personal contact with the clinic to which the patient is referred (Bender & Koshy, 1991; Brigg & Mudd, 1968; Cohen & Richardson, 1970; Ewalt, Cohen, & Harmatz, 1972; Frankel & Hovell, 1978; Jones & Hedley, 1988; Joshi et al., 1986), and lack of a sense of urgency in obtaining treatment (Campbell et al., 1991; Swenson & Pekarik, 1988) all have been found to be related to treatment noncompliance. A number of studies suggest that patients may be more likely to withdraw from treatment the longer the lag time between initial contact with the health or mental health system and initial treatment appointment (Axelrod & Wetzler, 1989; Backland & Lundwall, 1975; Bender & Koshy, 1991; Benjamin-Bauman, Reiss, & Bailey, 1984; Clarke, 1988; Frankel & Hovell, 1978; Mennicke, Lent, & Burgoyne, 1988; Raynes & Warren, 1971; Swenson & Pekarik, 1988).

Treatment noncompliance is widely considered problematic because of consequences such as inefficient use of staff time under conditions of increasing demand and dwindling clinical resources (Allan, 1988; Dubinsky, 1986; Palmer & Hampton, 1987), and because it results in lost revenues (Allan, 1988; Jones & Hedley, 1988; Palmer & Hampton, 1987). With regard to suicidal adolescents and others in need of speedy response by health and mental health agencies, there is also the concern that noncompliance increases the risk of self-injury, deteriorating health, or death (Jones & Hedley, 1988; Swenson & Pekarik, 1988).

Various methods have been employed in attempts to reduce treatment noncompliance. The following methods have been found to have an effect in reducing missed appointments. (See Macharia, Leon, Rowe, Stephenson, & Haynes, 1992, for a general overview.) Telephone reminders of appointments (Brigg & Mudd, 1968; Turner & Vernon, 1976; Vikander et al., 1986), mailed reminders (Kolko et al.,

1985; Nazarin et al., 1974; Swenson & Pekarik, 1988), questionnaires (Jones & Hedley, 1988; Joshi et al., 1986; Vikander et al., 1986), establishing personal contact with patients before intake to make them feel less anxious and/or better informed about treatment (Brigg & Mudd, 1968; Frankel & Hovell, 1978), active effort required on the part of the applicant (Joshi et al., 1986; Palmer & Hampton, 1987), and reduction of referral-to-appointment lag time (Benjamin-Bauman et al., 1984; Clarke, 1988; Frankel & Hovell, 1978; Joshi et al., 1986).

Several approaches are relevant to the procedure to be described in this chapter. Joshi and associates (1986) found that requiring parents to complete a questionnaire before attending appointments in a child psychiatric clinic significantly decreased broken appointments, or DNKs ("Did Not Keeps") from 35 percent to 9 percent, decreased referral-to-appointment lag time from 33 to 10 days, and increased the mean overall number of appointments kept from three to seven. Elsewhere, Palmer and Hampton (1987) reduced the DNK rate in a community mental health center from 38 percent to 15 percent by requiring clients to schedule an initial interview with the chief of the outpatient department before initiating treatment. In another study, Benjamin-Bauman and colleagues (1984) found that a lag time of less than one week led to significantly lower DNK rates than was true with a lag time of more than two weeks. Finally, Vikander and associates (1986) suggested overbooking of intake appointments as a method to reduce the negative effects of missed appointments on the efficiency of clinic functioning.

A MULTIFAMILY INTAKE GROUP

This chapter reports on the implementation of a multifamily intake group in an outpatient crisis intervention, brief treatment (6 to 12 weeks), and referral program for depressed and/or suicidal adolescents and their families in an inner-city area. This intake group was implemented for several reasons. First of all, there was a concern regarding detrimental effects of long referral-to-appointment lag times upon both the patient population and the functioning of the clinic. Second, there was a desire to implement a procedure that would incorporate several of the findings of other research, including the following: positive effects on patients of increased personal contact with clinic staff before the beginning of treatment; positive effects on patients of being informed about what to expect from treatment; usefulness of over-booking in reducing initial DNKs; and the effectiveness of reducing lag time in decreasing DNKs.

The intent of the intake group was to shorten or abolish the waiting list in the program, "weed out" patients and their parents who were not actually interested in treatment, and increase compliance with treatment. In addition, the intake group itself included: an introduction to the clinic, intended to familiarize patients and their families with what they should expect from treatment; a psychoeducational component to give adolescents and their parents a sense of what to do in case of an upsurge of suicidal ideation between clinic appointments; and a brief assessment of the current level of suicidal risk in the adolescents who attended the group, so that triage decisions could be made.

It was hoped that this procedure would significantly reduce lag time between referral and initial contact in the clinic, while also increasing compliance rates, as measured both by attendance at the initial clinic appointment and by continuation in treatment beyond two appointments. It was assumed that if the lag time between referral and first appointment was reduced, compliance with the initial intake appointment would increase. It was further assumed that the nature of this first appointment, which included a psychoeducational module, personal contact with clinic staff, and information about the clinic, would increase continued compliance with treatment beyond the first appointment.

In the following sections, we first provide some results of implementation of the multifamily intake group (known as the Orientation Group). Second, we describe the design of the group itself; in this latter section, we provide clinical examples of the process that typically occurred in the group.

RESULTS OF IMPLEMENTATION OF THE ORIENTATION GROUP

Compliance with referrals for treatment in the clinic was assessed using two groups of adolescents: Group 1 included 134 referrals preceding the implementation of the Orientation Group, and Group 2 was comprised of 75 adolescents who were referred after the intake group was implemented. Both groups included all adolescents judged appropriate for treatment in the clinic during a given period of time; there was no preselection of patients other than by the criterion of appropriateness for treatment. There were no significant differences between the groups in mean age, sex distribution, or ethnic/racial makeup. (See Zimmerman and Asnis, 1991a, for a more detailed presentation of the results of this study.)

Mean lag time between telephone screening and first appointment was reduced significantly, from 26 days for Group 1 to eight days for Group 2 ($t = 8.33$; df = 207; $p < .0001$). The percentage of adolescents who were noncompliers—that is, who never attended any appointments in the clinic—dropped from 49 percent of cases in Group 1 to 29 percent of Group 2 cases (Chi-square = 7.828; df = 1; $p = .005$). An additional 17 percent of Group 1 cases and 16 percent of Group 2 cases who attended the first appointment in the clinic withdrew before the third appointment. Thus, 66 percent of Group 1 and 45 percent of Group 2 were noncompliers or early dropouts; members of Group 2 were significantly less likely to be noncompliers or early dropouts (Chi-square = 10.516; df = 2; $p = .015$).

When continued compliance with treatment was examined, it was found that 78 percent of Group 1 compliers (i.e., those who attended one appointment) returned for a second appointment; this was true of 79 percent of Group 2 compliers.

The implementation of the multifamily intake group clearly succeeded in accomplishing some of its goals. First of all, referral-to-appointment lag time decreased substantially, from nearly one month to just over one week. The reduction of lag time was apparently a consequence of overbooking, since all patients referred to the clinic in a given week were invited to attend the group at the same time. This led to a reduced need to "chase after" patients and families who were unable or unwilling to attend their appointments, which allowed staff to be available more quickly for patients who were available for treatment.

A second way in which the implementation of the intake group was successful was in increasing patient compliance with the initial appointment in the clinic. The DNK rate of 49 percent preceding implementation of the intake group was at the high end of the range found in the literature; initial DNK rates of approximately 19 percent to 57 percent have been found in various studies (Benjamin-Bauman et al., 1984; Palmer & Hampton, 1987). Particularly in light of the high-risk profile of the population served by the clinic in the present study—

depressed and suicidal adolescents and their families—the decrease in this initial DNK rate to 29 percent is encouraging.

Our findings support the suggestion made by Vikander and associates (1986) that overbooking may be an effective way of reducing nonattendance at initial intake appointments; the current results also are consistent with those of Benjamin-Bauman and colleagues (1984), who maintained that a lag time of under one week should lead to significantly lower DNK rates as compared to a lag time of over two weeks.

Third, the implementation of the intake group in the current study increased the percentage of patients who were in treatment for more than two appointments, suggesting that the reduction of lag time also increased the likelihood of maintaining a high-risk population in treatment.

However, the intake group procedure was not found to have increased the likelihood that those who attended their first appointment would return for a second one. This finding does not confirm results reported by others that suggested that familiarity with clinic procedures, preadmission meetings with senior clinic staff, or the requirement of active effort to obtain treatment would increase the rate at which patients would return for further appointments (Brigg & Mudd, 1968; Frankel & Hovell, 1978; Joshi et al., 1986; Palmer & Hampton, 1987).

Since treatment follow-through is a complex phenomenon with patient, therapist, and clinic variables impinging upon it (Mennicke et al., 1988; Mohl, Martinez, Tichnor, & Appleby, 1989), it is unclear why the implementation of the Orientation Group did not increase the likelihood that patients would return for a second treatment session. It should be noted, however, that 78 percent of patients who attended their first appointment before the implementation of the group intake procedure returned for a second appointment, as compared with 79 percent of those who attended the Orientation Group. This is consistent with the findings of Weighill and associates (1983), who reported a rate of return for a second appointment of 78 percent. It is possible that this return rate is high enough so as to approach an asymptotic level for this population; that is, that compliance beyond approximately 80 percent may not occur under any circumstances.

Given the finding that the implementation of a multifamily intake group succeeded in decreasing referral-to-appointment lag time and in increasing initial compliance with treatment, the remainder of this chapter describes the process of the group itself. Relevant clinical examples illustrate various techniques and their effects on adolescents and their families during the outpatient clinic intake process.

THE PROCESS OF THE ORIENTATION GROUP

Referrals to the Group

In general, referrals to the clinic were taken by telephone, at which point a staff member determined whether a case appeared appropriate for the program. In cases deemed appropriate through telephone screening, patients and their parents or guardians were invited—by telephone with a confirmation by mail—to attend a weekly Orientation Group, scheduled on Wednesdays at 4 P.M. They were told that the process of registration and the group would take a total of about two hours to complete. Parents were informed that they would be required to attend this group before being assigned to a therapist for treatment in the clinic.

Completion of Forms

Preceding the group, the adolescent and family members registered for the clinic and began filling out assessment forms. These forms, which took approximately 60 to 75 minutes to complete, included demographic information, assessments of suicidality and homicidality in the adolescent and family members, checklists of current symptoms, and measures of family functioning, depression, aggression and impulsivity, and social desirability. (See Zimmerman and Asnis, 1991a, for a description of the instruments used.) The forms, completed both by adolescents and family members, were employed in several ways:

1. An immediate review of self-reported symptoms and functioning could be accomplished before the beginning of the Orientation Group, to be used to inform ad hoc triage decisions.
2. Comparisons could be made between the self-reports of the suicidal adolescents and family members, both to assess risk factors and to determine the degree of agreement or discrepancies between the reports. (See Zimmerman and Asnis, 1991b, for a discussion of such discrepancies.)

3. Data could be employed in other research projects in the clinic, subject to informed consent by the adolescent and family members.

Following the completion of the forms, adolescents and their family members were invited into the Orientation Group with other families who were referred to the clinic during the same time period.

Introductions and the Issue of Confidentiality

Upon entering the group, participants were introduced to the clinic staff in attendance. Immediately following, the issue of confidentiality was raised, and participants were asked to agree that they would keep the content of the meeting, as well as the identities of other participants, confidential. The group leader generally made this issue concrete and relevant to the lives of the participants, saying something like the following:

> If you were walking down the street tomorrow, and you saw Juan, who you met in the group today, you'd have to agree not to say "Hey, didn't I meet you in that group at the hospital for crazy teenagers yesterday?" Remember, some people feel uncomfortable about being here and don't want their business broadcast in the neighborhood.

The limits of confidentiality also were outlined: Participants were told that clinic staff would be required to report to authorities if an individual was at risk of harm to self or others, or if there was evidence of current physical or sexual abuse in the individual's household. In several years of operation of the Orientation Group, no participant refused to agree to keep the identity of participants or the content of the meeting confidential.

Following the explanation of confidentiality, participants were asked to introduce themselves, at least by first name. This request was made in order to reduce the formality of the group and to encourage participants to speak to each other as well as to the group leader. Frequently, participants gave more than their name, such as their relationship to other group members (e.g., mother to son, etc.), their reason for being in the group, and so on. The group leader also openly encouraged interchange among group members. This interchange sometimes was quite effective in conveying the experience of suicidal adolescents and their parents to each other.

Overview of the Clinic

Once introductions and an agreement regarding confidentiality were completed, the group leader presented a brief overview of the clinic and its functions. This overview included descriptions of the structure of the clinic, the evaluation process, active research protocols in the program, and the process of treatment in the clinic.

Structure of the Clinic

Participants in the Orientation Group were told that the clinic is a short-term, crisis-intervention, and brief treatment program for depressed and suicidal adolescents and their families. They also were told that at the end of treatment, referrals would be made to other mental health facilities as appropriate and that follow-up contacts would be made by clinic staff over the subsequent year. The evaluation process in the clinic then was explained to participants.

Evaluation Process

The explanation of the evaluation process was comprised of a discussion of self-report forms employed in the clinic, initial clinical interviews, neuropsychological screening, and research protocols. The rationale presented for employing *self-report forms* was that this method, in conjunction with other evaluation techniques, allowed for the rapid collection of a large amount of information. Participants were told that this was necessary in a brief-treatment, crisis-oriented program such as the one they were entering. They also were told that information from the forms would be useful in guiding subsequent clinical interviews and triage decisions. Finally, they were informed that the forms would be reviewed between the Orientation Group and the first appointment with the clinician assigned to their case, so that the clinician would not have to "start at the 'very beginning' all over again." Typically, adolescents and their families who had recently gone through scrutiny by a number of mental health professionals, in schools, hospitals, and other clinics, were visibly relieved at the thought that they would not have to tell their whole story once more from the "very beginning."

At times, participants had not completed the forms before the time of the group. In this case, they were told that they would need to come early to their next appointment in order to finish them. In addition, some participants were resistant to completing the forms.

Case Example

Mr. Johnson had brought his daughter, Liza, to the clinic after she had made a suicide attempt that had required brief hospitalization until she was medically stable. Mr. Johnson maintained that there was no reason for *him* to complete any forms, since he had not done anything to harm himself. The clinician overseeing the initial intake process explained to him that, even if he did nothing self-destructive, his daughter lived in his household, and her behavior must have affected him and his family. Moreover, he was told that it is generally the case that family events affect children deeply, so that information about the family was useful and important in helping his daughter understand and cope with the circumstances that led to her suicide attempt. Mr. Johnson then agreed to complete the forms for the sake of his daughter.

It should be noted that there were instances in which individuals, either adolescents or their family members, refused to complete the forms. In such instances, they were strongly encouraged to proceed, but no one was denied treatment in the clinic if forms were not completed. The philosophy of the clinic was that the cost of nonintervention in high-risk cases clearly outweighs the loss of information engendered by blank evaluation forms.

After an explanation of the use of self-report forms in the clinic, the process of the *initial clinical interviews* was outlined to participants in the Orientation Group. They were informed that these initial interviews with the clinician assigned to them would include a history-taking, an investigation of chronic risk factors, and inquiries about the current crisis and precipitating factors. They also were told that it was expected that parents would be involved in the process. Again, some families were resistant, either because they did not want to "rehash" recent disturbing, even harrowing, events or because they did not want to meet as a family about their difficulties.

Case Example

Ms. Suerto and her daughter, Alicia, appeared for the Orientation Group one week after Alicia had ingested a large and varied quantity of pills. Alicia had been kept in a hospital emergency room for several days until she was medically and psychiatrically stable enough to go home. In the Orientation Group, both mother and daughter maintained that everything was fine and that they did not have any problems now. The group leader confronted them on this; so did other participants in the group, who said that they found it hard to believe that "everything was fine" one week after Alicia's serious suicide attempt. At this, Ms. Suerto burst into tears and said that she didn't want to think about it any more because it was so awful and she felt extremely guilty, thinking it was her fault. The group leader empathized with her feelings and then pointed out that these feelings were a good reason why they *should* continue in treatment, so that such an awful situation would not recur. He also strongly supported the family's strength and potential for health, in that they had chosen to come to the clinic despite not wanting to revisit such disturbing feelings and frightening events. Subsequently, both Ms. Suerto and Alicia participated in treatment.

One advantage of having such interactions occur in a group setting is that participants can gain support both from the empathy of the clinician and from that of others who have experienced similar circumstances in their lives. Another advantage is that other participants can understand more clearly the rationale for and salience of family participation in treatment, as well as in the review of past history and events culminating in referral to the clinic.

Another approach frequently taken by the group leader to elucidate the need for history-taking and reconfrontation of the crisis was to present the model for intervention propounded by the clinic. Specifically, the group leader often said:

One reason we need to understand more from you about what has gone on in your lives and what happened that brought you to the clinic is that we are not mind-readers. Although we are trained experts in helping you to understand and cope with the events and feelings you have experienced recently, *you* are the experts on your own lives. In the beginning of your relationship with your therapist, we will need to learn from you about who you are, what has happened to you, and how you can find solutions so that such things won't happen again. You will be the teachers, we will be the students. Even later on, we will work with you like a team: We will try to help you to improve your situation yourselves, rather than tell you what to do. That way, when you leave the clinic, you are more likely to have methods and approaches to future problems that will work, because you will have developed them yourselves, with the assistance of our expertise.

This speech, or a variant of it, was offered to make clear the collaborative nature of treatment in the clinic and to enlist the ego and family resources of prospective patients.

Active Research Protocols

The third aspect of the presentation in the Orientation Group about the evaluation process in the clinic was a description of a *neuropsychological screening battery* that had been designed and implemented in the clinic, followed by a discussion of ongoing *research protocols* in which patients might participate on a voluntary basis. The details of these two components of clinic functioning are not directly pertinent to the content of this chapter, but are described extensively elsewhere. (See Zimmerman, 1993, for a description of the neuropsychological screening, and Grosz et al., 1990a, 1990b, for a description of biological research projects carried out in the clinic.)

Process of Treatment in the Clinic

Following a description of the evaluation process, the process of psychotherapy in the clinic was presented to participants in the Orientation Group. This part of the presentation included a discussion of goals of treatment, modalities offered, fee policies, frequency of appointments, and expectations regarding who should attend appointments.

Participants were told that there were several goals of treatment in the clinic. Initially, treatment would focus on *stabilization*—not only with regard to acute symptoms the adolescent was experiencing, but also with regard to the potential for impulsive action on his or her part. Further, it was explained that stabilization of the family would be addressed, in relation to reactions to the behavior of the adolescent as well as to chronic areas of dysfunction. Here again, some parents were resistant to the idea of participating in treatment; the group leader would then reinforce the idea that an adolescent's behavior strongly affects the family, while family functioning also has a powerful influence on the behavior of the adolescent.

A second general goal of treatment in the clinic was a deepened *understanding of suicidal behavior.* Participants in the Orientation Group were told that this process would begin in the group itself, in that there would be a discussion of what to do when a person seems depressed or suicidal. (See "Psychoeducational Module," which follows.)

A third goal of treatment was *improved individual and school or vocational functioning* for the adolescent as well as improved functioning of the family as a whole. In this context, the group leader suggested that as the adolescent strove toward more independent, adult functioning, internally and in school, work, and interpersonal spheres, more effective family functioning would help support him or her in this effort. Succinctly, if the family was cohesive, this would help the adolescent to move beyond the sphere of the family into the adult world.

Next, the forms and philosophy of treatment were described briefly to group participants. They were told that since the clinic held to a crisis intervention and brief treatment model, an integrative approach was taken; that is, that several modalities would be offered simultaneously, and that technical approaches employed would be dictated by the needs of each individual case. Typically, treatment would include individual sessions for the adolescent and family sessions, both provided by the same clinician; in some cases, separate appointments for a parent and/ or other family members would be appropriate as well. Often, cognitive-behavioral interventions were structured into the treatment when specific issues arose; these generally included exercises designed to promote more open and supportive family communication, clearer definition of responsibilities within the family, and the development of more effective parenting skills.

The modalities provided would depend on the nature of the issues with which the adolescent and family were struggling; the rationale given for this approach was that it allowed for greater leverage in a short period of time. Frequently, the question of preservation of confidentiality arose in this context: Adolescents were concerned about having their parents know things that they did not want them to know; parents sometimes expressed similar concerns. The group leader would then explain that confidentiality would be maintained, subject to the limits described earlier in the group. (See "Introductions and the Issue of Confidentiality" earlier.) Further, participants were told the following:

> There may be times when one of you will tell your therapist something that he or she believes should be talked about with other family members. For example, you [gesturing to a parent] might believe that your child is using drugs, or you [nodding to an adolescent] might feel that your parent's anger is making you feel suicidal. In such a case, the therapist may offer to help you discuss the issue with other family members; however, unless you are a danger to yourself or others, the therapist will not speak up if you insist. On the other hand, there may be times when the therapist will tell you that therapy is being seriously hindered if this issue cannot be discussed and will strongly encourage you to bring it up with his or her support.

It was rare that such issues arose without being addressed later in family sessions. Occasionally, however, the therapist was compelled to say that therapy could not proceed unless a given issue was addressed more openly. In most cases, this led to an airing of the problem at hand, generally with positive results.

Case Example

Annie was a 17-year-old girl who had made a serious suicide attempt with an overdose of medication. Subsequently, she tried to "put on a happy face" with her family. Her mother was a harsh, often unempathic woman prone to angry outbursts in the family; she herself also had threatened suicide in earlier years when confronted by her husband or children over her behavior. Annie continued to be somewhat depressed, but did not want to reveal this to her mother for fear that her mother would become enraged or suicidal herself. With the therapist's encouragement, she spoke with her mother in a family session about her feelings. Although her mother began to cry, she also was able to say that she did not want Annie to keep such things from her, since she loved Annie and did not want to lose her. Mother and daughter, along with other family members, then were able to talk more openly about how Annie could feel more supported and less isolated from the family. Annie's mother ultimately asked for a referral for treatment for herself upon discharge from the clinic.

Following the discussion of treatment modalities, participants were told that fees were based on ability to pay and that Medicaid coverage would be accepted. They were also told:

> When we schedule an appointment, we assume that you will be able to make the appointment unless you let us know more than a day in advance that you can't come. If you cancel without advance notice, or you simply don't show up for your appointment, we will expect you to pay for the appointment. This is because we take our work and your problems seriously, and we expect you to do the same.

Participants were asked to sign a copy of the Fees and Appointments Policy, and were given a copy to take with them. They also were given the general clinic telephone number and were told that they would have a number for their therapist as soon as he or she was assigned to them.

In general, sessions were scheduled for twice per week; once for the adolescent alone and once for the family (including the adolescent). Again, the vicissitudes of each given case were taken into account in scheduling, such as the patient's and family's availability and their need for and ability to tolerate a recommended intensity of treatment.

The group leader made it clear to participants in the Orientation Group that the clinic strongly recommended that the adolescent and available family members be fully involved in treatment. As is apparent from the statement given earlier, attendance was treated as a contractual matter as much as possible. In another sense, this contract was made explicit by stating that the clinic would offer expertise in helping the adolescent and family to resolve difficult issues and improve overall functioning, while the staff would expect the adolescent and family to be as fully committed as possible to working on the issues that arose. In the Orientation Group, it was emphasized that this commitment would include attendance at scheduled appointments and support of treatment goals.

Psychoeducational Module

Subsequent to these descriptions of clinic procedures and the evaluation and treatment process, the group leader presented a psychoeducational module on adolescent suicide. This interactive module included: the distinction between suicidal ideation and a suicide attempt; problem-solving alternatives; effective communication; and contracting. There were specific goals to be accomplished during each component.

Suicidal Ideation and Suicide Attempts

Participants initially were introduced to the basic distinction among thoughts, feelings, and actions. They were asked to define each, and the group leader clarified the differences—particularly between thoughts and feelings on the one hand and actions on the other. The goal to be accomplished was to help adolescents and their parents understand that many adolescents experience suicidal ideation and that preventing all suicidal ideation may be a daunting task; on the other hand, it was made clear that taking actual self-destructive action was less common and more serious, and that adolescents and their parents could take specific steps to prevent such action.

The leader then presented a brief overview of some research regarding suicidal ideation and attempts in adolescence:

Every year, about 5,000 adolescents take their own lives in this country. Does that sound like too many? [Participants generally agree that it does.] In this clinic, we feel that even one adolescent suicide is too many, since teenagers rarely really want to die—at least, not without ambivalence—and their self-destructive behavior is frequently a misguided attempt to solve a problem rather than end their lives. In addition, research estimates that there are 50 to 100 attempts for every completed suicide, meaning that 250,000 to 500,000 adolescents make suicide attempts per year. This shows you that it is a large, serious problem in the United States.

Now, how many adolescents do you think have *thought* about killing themselves at some time or another? [Answers range widely, although adolescents themselves generally state that most teenagers think about suicide.] In research done in a New York

City high school, 62 percent of adolescents who completed an anonymous survey reported having thought about suicide at some time in their lives. In addition, about 8 percent of them reported actually making a suicide attempt. [See Harkavy Friedman, Asnis, Boeck, and DiFiore, 1987, and Zimmerman and Morledge, 1992, for more information about these studies.] That means that five out of eight—more than half of the high school students in the research—reported suicidal thoughts, and one of every 12 or 13 actually acted on their thoughts.

This shows two things: First of all, many adolescents think about suicide; it is a fairly common, although certainly painful, experience. Second, a smaller percentage, but still too many, make suicide attempts. It is good to know that not all teenagers who think about suicide also make a suicide attempt, because that allows others to help them before they do such a self-harmful thing. This is one of the things we try to work on with you in this clinic: We try to help you break the link in the chain between thinking about suicide and acting on your thoughts.

So, let's talk about it for a minute: Why do adolescents try to kill themselves, to end their lives? [The group leader then would solicit responses from participants. Generally, these included such reasons as a breakup with a boy- or girlfriend; arguments with parents; school failure; anger; depression; and so on. Participants, on their own, frequently identified precipitants such as these, which also often have been reported in research on adolescent suicide. [See, for example, Alcohol, Drug Abuse, and Mental Health Administration, 1989; Pfeffer, 1989b.]]

Problem-Solving Alternatives

At this point, when the magnitude of the problem of adolescent suicidality had been presented and some discussion of precipitants had been initiated, the group leader moved on toward assisting participants in considering and developing alternatives to suicidal behavior. The goal of this component of the psychoeducational model was to help adolescents to consider options they may have when feeling suicidal. The intent was to indicate that, if actions other than suicidal behavior could be substituted, the suicidal thoughts and feelings might well subside and the adolescent would be glad not to have taken self-destructive action.

The simple question posed to the group was: "What can someone who is feeling suicidal do instead of trying to end his or her life? What can you do next time instead of doing something self-destructive?" Each adolescent in the group was asked to respond in turn, and these responses were employed both as ways to develop problem-solving alternatives and as a triage method for the group leader. When individuals were not responsive, either out of discomfort with speaking in a large group or because of resistance to the group process, they were asked to stay after the group for an individual assessment and triage decision.

Case Example

Maria, who had made a suicide attempt by overdose of prescription medication, sat next to her mother; the two exchanged few glances during the group and appeared somewhat resistant to the process. However, in answer to the preceding question, Maria said that she could tell her mother when she was feeling suicidal. At this, her mother burst into tears, and Maria admitted that she realized how much her mother cared about her as a result of discussions they had had in the hospital emergency room after her suicide attempt. She acknowledged that she now felt she could turn to her mother for support and that her mother would understand.

Case Example

Jonas, who had cut his wrist with a box cutter, said that he could call a friend if he felt suicidal. When asked what his friend would say or do, Jonas said: "He'd say, 'What do you want to do a stupid thing like that for?!'" Questioned about how this would make him feel, Jonas responded that this would remind him that he did not want to end his life and that he would feel his friend's support. He also said that listening to music or taking a walk sometimes helped reduce his level of suicidality.

Case Example

Antoinette attended the Orientation Group alone. She was 18 years old and stated that her mother was not interested in coming. She also had a history of several suicide attempts with various methods. When asked what she could do next time instead of trying to take her own life, she responded: "I could imagine myself lying in my coffin, and seeing all my friends and family around, being sorry that I was dead. I would look beautiful and peaceful in the coffin." She could not articulate how this fantasy would help reduce her suicidal thoughts and urges.

These three examples describe well the range of responses to the question of what one can do instead of acting upon suicidal impulses. Maria's response is clearly the most hopeful, in that she would have someone close at hand upon whom she could perhaps rely. However, the question still arises as to why she could not reach out to her mother in the past and if this change of heart is in fact strong, solid, and realistic. Given a statement like Maria's—and her mother's reaction—the group leader would then reinforce the importance of having someone to go to for support; however, the salience of being able to express the need for this support would also be emphasized.

Jonas's situation is perhaps a bit more problematic, in that he appeared to gain support from his friend's response, but his friend's words were somewhat pejorative in tone. This is not unusual in the reactions of others to expressions of suicidal ideation in adolescence. Many people respond by attempting to talk the adolescent out of his or her feelings, or by deriding the teenager for having the impulses in the first place. The difficulty here is that, although some adolescents feel support in this approach—and it frequently gives voice to one combatant in their own internal battle regarding suicidal ideation—it is not particularly empathic with the adolescent's feelings of isolation, desperation, and pain. Further, it sides explicitly with the adolescent's own self-deprecatory thoughts, and this ultimately can increase suicidal ideation in some individuals.

In addition, Jonas expressed the idea that listening to music and taking a walk were helpful to him in containing his suicidal impulses. Many adolescents made similar statements about their management of thoughts and feelings, also mentioning other activities such as exercise, watching TV, sleeping, and sometimes crying as well. These other activities were by no means discouraged, although participants in the Orientation Group were encouraged to consider to which family members, friends, or figures in the community (members of the clergy, teachers, etc.) they might turn for support. It was emphasized that support and contact with other people is often a stronger deterrent to suicidal acting out than are other methods. Nevertheless, the group leader underscored the importance of having *some* method available to "break the link in the chain between suicidal thoughts and actions," so that adolescents feel that they have some increased ability to attenuate their self-destructive impulses.

Finally, Antoinette's statement is included here because there are some cases in which it is clear at intake that some immediate intervention must be taken. Antoinette had a well-developed fantasy of her death, had scant support from others in her life, was a repeat suicide attempter, and had little ability to demonstrate alternatives to suicidal behavior through problem-solving or impulse control. These are all hallmarks of individuals at high risk for suicidal behavior and eventual completed suicide (Holinger, 1989; Pfeffer, 1989a). Immediately after the group, she was escorted to the hospital emergency room to be assessed for admission to a psychiatric inpatient unit.

Effective Communication

Typically, the process of the Orientation Group evolved naturally from a discussion of alternatives to suicidal behavior to how adolescents and their parents might communicate more effectively, with the goal in mind that self-destructive patterns would be attenuated. In essence, the consideration of the subject of effective communication included three aspects: With whom does the adolescent feel comfortable enough to reach out for support? What are effective ways for parents to talk and listen to their suicidal adolescent? What do adolescents need when they are feeling suicidal?

The range of people to whom adolescents felt they could turn for support was extensive, including parents, siblings, other family members, friends, and professionals in the community. Stressed as salient in the Orientation Group were both the adolescent's ability to reach out and the other person's ability to respond appropriately and in such a way as to attenuate the intensity of the adolescent's current crisis. Typically, the group leader asked, "Who can you turn to when you feel suicidal?" and then, "How do you want [the person] to respond to you? What will make you feel better?"

Many adolescents stated that what they seek is a sense that the individual to whom they turn in moments of suicidal crisis understands what they are going through and can withstand the intensity of their emotions.

Case Example

Angelina said that she could turn to her aunt, ten years her senior, but not to her mother. She said that her aunt could relate to what she was feeling and could sit with her and listen; her mother, by contrast, would become anxious and tearful and ask her what she (her mother) was doing wrong. Angelina made it clear that her mother's reaction made her feel more alone and guilty that she was causing her mother suffering; this increased her suicidal ideation. She also said that her mother's reaction made her angry, because her mother was thinking more of herself than of Angelina's pain. Her mother's response made Angelina feel that she should not be feeling the way she was and made her less able to think through possible alternatives to suicidal behavior; her aunt's response gave her the sense that there was someone who could tolerate the intensity of the feelings without "crumbling." This knowledge, that someone could hear her pain and bear to listen to it without her own agenda, was comforting to Angelina and helped alleviate her crisis.

Although most adolescents sought the kind of response exemplified by Angelina's aunt, some expressed the need for a more aggressive stance by others toward their suicidality. Jonas, described earlier, was one individual for whom this kind of stance appeared ameliorative. In another case, Tonya said that she became less suicidal when her mother reminded her that she had "so much to live for" and that she had talents and abilities that would be wasted if she killed herself. Some adolescents also maintained that their suicidal impulses decreased when someone pointed out the effect their death would have on others.

Case Example

Robert stated that he told his mother that he had thoughts of ending his life, to which she responded, "How could you do such a thing to me?" This made Robert stop and think about the consequences of his contemplated act on her and others around him—his younger sister, his girlfriend, and so on—and he chose not to take any self-destructive action as a result.

Such approaches, which appeal to the adolescent's sense of responsibility to others or to his or her own future, sometimes are effective in attenuating suicidal impulses and therefore reducing the likelihood of an untimely death. They make explicit the potential manipulative component of suicidal behavior ("You'll be sorry when I'm dead") and compel adolescents to be aware of their importance to others and the effect their death would have. However, they also are somewhat problematic in many cases, since they may lead the adolescent to feel guilty about suicidal feelings or overly responsible for the welfare of others. In turn, these feelings may ultimately *potentiate* suicidal impulses rather than attenuate them, since the adolescent may identify internally with the "aggressor" and feel the need for self-punishment (Zimmerman, 1991). Consequently, adolescents and their family members who attended the Orientation Group were encouraged to learn to relate and respond to each other in more sensitive, straightforwardly supportive ways.

With this in mind, the group leader presented some fundamental elements of effective listening. Adolescents and their family members were told that most people need someone to listen and respond as did Angelina's aunt, with empathy and with a relatively sanguine reaction to expressions of suicidal thoughts and impulses. It was emphasized that this did not mean that others should ignore a suicidal adolescent or treat his or her feelings and thoughts as insignificant or not serious. Quite to the contrary, the group leader emphasized consistently the seriousness and potential dangerousness of suicidal thoughts and impulses in adolescents, underlining the adolescent's need for others to respond in kind but without being overly anxious, angry, or punitive. To the point, the group leader frequently said some variant of the following:

What is important to understand is that suicidal teenagers need to feel that someone is trying to understand them, the way they are and how they feel at that moment. They do not usually want someone to talk them out of their feelings, make them feel guilty, or fall apart in front of them. In fact, many times they don't want someone who talks at all; they need someone who can listen without getting too upset and who can make them feel supported. Sometimes this means just sitting there and letting your teenager talk to you without making any responses at all, except maybe to say something like "That must hurt a lot" or "What do you need me to do to help?"

Although the suggestion that someone could be effective by behaving this way is not foreign to many mental health professionals, it often seemed silly or impotent to the parents of suicidal adolescents, who themselves were suffering indirectly with their child's pain. However, within the context of the Orientation Group, adolescents frequently lent support and credence to the group leader's statement; this, in turn, made their parents agree to attempt to take such a stance when suicidality next arose in their child.

Contracting

An informal contract regarding suicidal behavior was next made between the adolescents in the Orientation Group, their families, and the group leader. This was implemented as a way of summarizing the content of the psychoeducational model presented in the Orientation Group, as a triage technique, and as a potential deterrent to further suicidal behavior.

The organizing principle of the contract made in the Orientation Group was simple: Adolescents were asked to outline a sequence of behaviors they would put into effect the next time they felt suicidal instead of committing a self-destructive act. Each adolescent in the group was asked in turn to do this, with the understanding that this was a form of preventive problem-solving. They were encouraged to include a list of things they could do, beginning with the one most likely to be effective in attenuating the intensity of their feelings. In most cases, the action at the top of the list was to contact a given individual whom they felt would be able to respond in an empathic way. Typically, individuals at the top of the adolescents' lists included parents, other family members, friends, teachers, and guidance counselors. Following this were activities such as those mentioned earlier—taking walks, exercising, listening to music, watching TV, drawing, writing, and so on.

Once adolescents had generated their plan, they and their families were told that, in addition to the resources they had listed for themselves, they also could telephone the clinic during weekday hours or go to a local hospital emergency room at other times.

The triage function of contracting was this: If adolescents were unable to generate a plan, or if their plan was indicative of little capacity to consider alternatives to suicidal behavior—as was the case with Antoinette, described earlier—they were asked to wait after the Orientation Group. The group leader then was able to meet individually with these adolescents and their family members, and make a determination of what next steps needed to be taken to assure that the adolescent would be safe.

Ending the Orientation Group

In concluding the Orientation Group, the group leader asked if there were any questions. This allowed for a review of material that had not been fully understood by participants; further, those with continued concern for their own immediate safety (or that of their child) could make this known at that time. Finally, participants were told that they would receive a telephone call within a short period of time from the clinician who would become their therapist. They also were informed that they could telephone the clinic in the interim and ask for the staff member on call if the need arose. In addition, they were given a brochure that described the clinic and provided some information about adolescent suicide, including signs and symptoms and what actions could be taken to prevent suicide attempts.

GUIDELINES FOR GROUP LEADERSHIP

Given the fact that the Orientation Group was a one-time, psychoeducational session with a high-risk population, a list of guidelines for leadership of such a group is offered here.

1. The provision of immediate evaluation is essential when an adolescent's level of risk appears too high. Thus, such a group is best held in a medical setting in which triage decisions can include the availability of emergent consideration for hospitalization. It is also best to have two staff members colead the group, so that one can be available for emergent response when necessary. In the case of the Orientation Group, one staff member was a trainee, and this helped introduce such individuals to the process of intervention with high-risk patients in a relatively contained setting.

2. Although the group should be structured clearly, including the provision to participants of an agenda at the outset, the time required for each module and subcomponent of the group should be flexible. This enables the leader to take into account the specific needs of a given group of individuals without losing sight of the overall objectives that must be accomplished in a certain period of time. Thus, although the group typically lasted approximately 45 to 60 minutes, the subcomponents would vary by as much as five minutes one way or the other to accommodate the needs of participants.

3. Within this flexible structure, however, limits must be placed on the interaction at times. It is not productive for one participant to monopolize the group's time, nor is it useful (or appropriate) for two or three participants (e.g., an adolescent and her parents) to engage in a high-intensity disagreement in the group. In order to prevent such interactions from leading the group astray, the leader must exert empathic but firm guidance, suggesting that such issues or interactions can be continued separately with a clinic staff member, either after the group or at the next appointment.

4. At times, because of the high-risk and sometimes unpredictable nature of a population such as suicidal adolescents and their parents, the leader may be drawn in by the intensity of the problems of a given participant or may find overpowering countertransference issues arising. Such difficulties, which threaten to overwhelm the personal resources of the leader, provide further impetus to the creation of a framework for the group that includes coleadership, firm structure and limits, and the triage backup of a hospital emergency room or other similar facility. It is not recommended that a group such as the Orientation Group be instituted in a setting that does not have support systems for the clinicians involved.

CONCLUSION

The multifamily intake described in this chapter was developed in order to respond rapidly to the needs of suicidal adolescents and their families. The Orientation Group was designed to meet the needs of this at-risk population in a number of ways: First of all, as is well documented in the literature, adolescent suicide attempters frequently are noncompliant with treatment, especially as the time between referral for treatment and the initial treatment appointment lengthens (Clarke,

1988; Rotheram-Borus, 1990; Swedo, 1989; Trautman & Rotheram, 1986). Since the Orientation Group allowed for a rapid response, some adolescents could be brought into treatment during a suicidal crisis but before they had actually committed a self-destructive act. In cases where a suicide attempt had already occurred, the intensity of stressors leading to the suicidal behavior could be acknowledged and addressed while the adolescents and their families were still accessible to treatment.

Second, the Orientation Group met the needs of suicidal adolescents and their families by providing a psychoeducational module that assisted them in managing suicidal behavior in both preventive and postventive ways. Regarding postvention, adolescents and their families took strides toward greater understanding of the etiology of suicidality and increased empathy with each other's experience of past events. Preventively, they became more aware of their problem-solving capacities in relation to the potential recurrence of suicidal thoughts and actions, and began to improve their ability to communicate in ways that would be more effective in reducing the likelihood of this recurrence.

Third, the rapid response made possible by the Orientation Group allowed clinical staff to assess adolescents and make triage decisions during or soon after the occurrence of a suicidal crisis. This also served a preventive and postventive function in that adolescents were less likely to be in crisis with no access to mental health services that could address their stressors and alleviate their emotional turmoil.

Finally, by providing an intake that included personal contact with clinic staff, the completion of evaluation forms, and active participation in a group format, the Orientation Group allowed adolescents and their families to develop a clearer sense of what they would experience in psychotherapy. For many of them, this made the transition from other mental health settings to the clinic, as well as the transition into treatment, more manageable, comprehensible, and familiar. In essence, they felt supported in coping with suicidality and in navigating the systems through which psychotherapy is provided in an urban setting. In a number of cases, adolescents and/or their parents later told clinic staff that the Orientation Group itself was therapeutic and led them to feel more committed to the hard work of reorienting their lives toward more effective and adaptive functioning.

REFERENCES

Adebonojo, F. O. (1973). A comparative study of child health care in urban and suburban children. *Clinical Pediatrics, 12,* 644–648.

Alcohol, Drug Abuse, and Mental Health Administration (1989). *Report of the Secretary's Task Force on youth suicide.* (U.S. Department of Health and Human Services Publication #[ADM]89-1621.) Washington, DC: Superintendent of Documents, U.S. Government Printing Office.

Allan, A. T. (1988). No-shows at a community mental health clinic: A pilot study. *International Journal of Social Psychiatry, 34*(1), 40–46.

Alpert, J. J. (1964). Broken appointments. *Pediatrics, 14,* 127–132.

Axelrod, S., & Wetzler, S. (1989). Factors associated with better compliance with psychiatric aftercare. *Hospital & Community Psychiatry, 40*(4), 397–401.

Backland, F., & Lundwall, L. (1975). Dropping out of treatment: A critical review. *Psychological Bulletin, 82*(5), 738–783.

Badgley, R. F., & Furnal, M. A. (1961). Appointment breaking in a pediatric clinic. *Yale Journal of Biology & Medicine, 34,* 117–123.

Bender, K. G., & Koshy, M. K. (1991). Returning for follow-up: Attendance compliance in an Indian psychiatric clinic. *International Journal of Social Psychiatry, 37*(3), 173–181.

Benjamin-Bauman, J., Reiss, M. L., & Bailey, J. S. (1984). Increasing appointment keeping by reducing the call-appointment interval. *Journal of Applied Behavioral Analysis, 17*(3), 295–301.

Brigg, E. H., & Mudd, E. H. (1968). An exploration of methods to reduce broken first appointments. *Family Coordinator, 17,* 41–46.

Campbell, B., Staley, D., & Matas, M. (1991). Who misses appointments? An empirical analysis. *Canadian Journal of Psychiatry, 36*(3), 223–225.

Cavanaugh, R. M. (1990). Utilizing the phone appointment for adolescent follow-up. *Clinical Pediatrics, 29*(6), 302–304.

Clarke, C. F. (1988). Deliberate self-poisoning in adolescents. *Archives of Disorders of Childhood, 63,* 1479–1483.

Cohen, R., & Richardson, C. (1970). A retrospective study of case attrition in a child psychiatry clinic. *Social Psychiatry, 5,* 77–83.

Dubinsky, M. (1986). Predictors of appointment non-compliance in community mental health patients. *Community Mental Health Journal, 22*(2), 142–146.

Ewalt, P., Cohen, M., & Harmatz, J. (1972). Prediction of treatment acceptance by child guidance clinic applicants: An easily applied instrument. *American Journal of Orthopsychiatry, 42,* 857–864.

Frankel, B. S., & Hovell, M. F. (1978). Health service appointment keeping: A behavioral view and critical review. *Behavioral Modification, 2,* 435–464.

Grosz, D., Asnis, G. M., Harkavy Friedman, J. M., Kausar, S., Zimmerman, J. K., & van Praag, H. M. (1990a, October). *The fenfluramine challenge in depressed adolescents.* Paper presented at the Annual Conference of the American Academy of Child and Adolescent Psychiatry, Chicago, IL.

Grosz, D., Asnis, G. M., Harkavy Friedman, J. M., Kausar, S., Zimmerman, J. K., & van Praag, H. M. (1990b, October). *Serotonergic responsivity in suicidal adolescents.* Paper presented at the Annual Conference of the American Academy of Child and Adolescent Psychiatry, Chicago, IL.

Harkavy Friedman, J. M., Asnis, G. M., Boeck, M., & DiFiore, J. (1987). Prevalence of specific suicidal behaviors in a high school sample. *American Journal of Psychiatry, 144*(9), 1203–1206.

Holinger, P. (1989). Epidemiologic issues in youth suicide. In C. R. Pfeffer (Ed.), *Suicide among youth: Perspectives on risk and prevention* (pp. 41–62). Washington, DC: American Psychiatric Association Press.

Jones, R. B., & Hedley, A. J. (1988). Reducing non-attendance in an outpatient clinic. *Public Health, 102,* 385–391.

Joshi, P. K., Maisami, M., & Coyle, J. T. (1986). Prospective study of intake procedures in a child psychiatry clinic. *Journal of Clinical Psychiatry, 47,* 111–113.

Kolko, D. J., Parrish, J. M., & Wilson, F. E. (1985). Obstacles to appointment keeping in a child behavior management clinic. *Child & Family Behavior Therapy, 7*(1), 9–15.

Macharia, W. M., Leon, G., Rowe, B. H., Stephenson, B. J., & Haynes, B. (1992). An overview of interventions to improve compliance with appointment keeping for medical services. *Journal of the American Medical Association, 267*(13), 1813–1817.

Mennicke, S. A., Lent, R. W., & Burgoyne, K. L. (1988). Premature termination from university counseling centers: A review. *Journal of Counseling & Development, 66*(10), 458–465.

Mohl, P. C., Martinez, E., Tichnor, J. G., & Appleby, A. (1989). Psychotherapy refusers. *Comprehensive Psychiatry, 30*(3), 245–250.

National Center for Health Statistics (1992). Advance report of final mortality statistics, 1989. *NCHS Monthly Vital Statistics Report, 40*(8, Suppl. 2).

Nazarin, L. F., Mechaber, J., Charney, E., & Coulter, M. P. (1974). Effects of a mailed appointment reminder on appointment keeping. *Pediatrics, 53,* 349–352.

Palmer, D., & Hampton, P. T. (1987). Reducing broken appointments at intake in a community mental health center. *Community Mental Health Journal, 23*(1), 76–78.

Pfeffer, C. R. (1989a). Life stress and family risk factors for youth fatal and nonfatal suicidal behavior. In C. R. Pfeffer (Ed.), *Suicide among youth:*

Perspectives on risk and prevention (pp. 143–164). Washington, DC: American Psychiatric Association Press.

Pfeffer, C. R. (Ed.) (1989b). *Suicide among youth: Perspectives on risk and prevention.* Washington, DC: American Psychiatric Association Press.

Raynes, A., & Warren, G. (1971). Some distinguishing features of patients failing to attend a psychiatric clinic after referral. *American Journal of Orthopsychiatry, 41,* 581–588.

Rotheram-Borus, M. J. (1990, October). *The treatment of adolescents who have attempted suicide.* Institute presentation at the Annual Meeting of the American Academy of Child and Adolescent Psychiatry, Chicago, IL.

Swedo, S. E. (1989). Postdischarge therapy of hospitalized adolescent suicide attempters. *Journal of Adolescent Health Care, 10,* 541–544.

Swenson, T. R., & Pekarik, G. (1988). Interventions for reducing missed initial appointments at a community mental health center. *Community Mental Health Journal, 24*(3), 205–218.

Trautman, P. D., & Rotheram, M. J. (1986, October). *Referral failure among adolescent suicide attempters.* Poster presented at the Annual Meeting of the American Academy of Child Psychiatry, Los Angeles, CA.

Turner, A. J., & Vernon, J. C. (1976). Prompts to increase attendance in a community mental health center. *Journal of Applied Behavioral Analysis, 9*(2), 141–145.

Vikander, T., Parnicky, K., Demers, R., Frisof, K., Demers, P., & Chase, N. (1986). New-patient no-shows in an urban family practice center: Analysis and intervention. *Journal of Family Practice, 22*(3), 263–268.

Weighill, V. E., Hodge, J., & Peck, D. F. (1983). Keeping appointments with clinical psychologists. *British Journal of Clinical Psychology, 22,* 143–144.

Zimmerman, J. K. (1991). Crossing the desert alone: An etiological model of female adolescent suicidality. In C. Gilligan, A. G. Rogers, & D. L. Tolman (Eds.), *Women, girls, & psychotherapy: Reframing resistance* (pp. 223–240). New York: Haworth Press.

Zimmerman, J. K. (1993, April). *The development of a brief neuropsychological screening battery.* Paper presented at the 26th Annual Conference of the American Association of Suicidology. San Francisco, CA.

Zimmerman, J. K., & Asnis, G. M. (1991a, August). *A multifamily intake group in a program for suicidal adolescents.* Paper presented at the 99th Annual Convention of the American Psychological Association, San Francisco, CA.

Zimmerman, J. K., & Asnis, G. M. (1991b). Parents' knowledge of children's suicide attempts. *American Journal of Psychiatry, 148*(8), 1091–1092.

Zimmerman, J. K., & Morledge, J. (1992). *Prevalence of specific suicidal behaviors in a high school sample: A replication and extension.* Unpublished manuscript.

PART III
Treatment

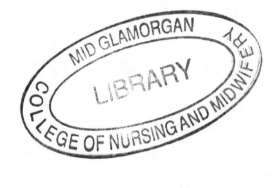

7

Psychodynamic Treatment of Adolescent Suicide Attempters

DAVID A. JOBES

Case Example

Mark was a depressed 19-year-old college freshman who was brought to the emergency room by a former high school coach after sustaining a superficial self-inflicted gunshot wound to the head. His depression and suicide attempt were apparently linked to a four-year homosexual relationship with his coach. Mark reported that while he had grown to love his coach, he hated their sexual involvement. He had come to feel trapped in the relationship, literally unable to live with him or without him. Upon his arrival home for spring break, Mark arranged to meet the coach in a park where they often met and had sexual encounters. When the coach arrived, he witnessed Mark put his father's handgun to his head. Fortunately, Mark turned the discharging gun away as he pulled the trigger. When asked why he had staged this attempt in front of his coach, Mark responded, ". . . it was payback time . . . I wanted to get him back and hurt him as much as he's hurt me . . . I could have ended my pain and his would have just begun."

OVERVIEW

The case of Mark dramatically reflects fundamental features of classic psychoanalytic thinking about suicide. This chapter examines these and other constructs related to suicide, specifically adolescent suicide, within a lineage of work that has evolved from Sigmund Freud and others in the psychoanalytic tradition. To address more fully various aspects of the topic, some psychodynamic theoretical perspectives and relevant research themes are discussed briefly prior to a fuller consideration of psychodynamic clinical interventions with suicidal teenagers.

THEORETICAL CONSIDERATIONS

The following is a brief review of some the major dynamic theoretical approaches to suicide and adolescent development.

Classic Psychoanalytic

Freud did not write at length about suicide specifically, but he did see a number of suicidal patients and provided some valuable perspectives. Freud's (1917/1957) classic work "Mourning and Melancholia" outlined the psychological mechanisms involved in turning hostility against the self, which explains the self-reproach/hate seen in suicidal (melancholic) depressions. As summarized by Shneidman (1980), the central Freudian position on suicide is that it represents murder in the 180th degree. Since people identify with and internalize the objects of their love with ambivalence, they may direct their own aggressive impulses against the internalized love object whom they both love and hate (e.g., the dynamic seen in the case of Mark). While retroflex rage was primary to Freud's thinking on the topic, suicide also could be conceptualized as an expression of the death instinct—a primary instinctual force in all living matter to return to a completely inert state (Freud, 1920/1955).

Karl Menninger's more direct and extensive consideration of suicide represented an important elaboration and extension of some of Freud's ideas. In his classic text, *Man Against Himself,* Menninger (1938) delineated analytic perspectives on hostility and the death instinct. Most notably, Menninger explained the psychodynamics of hostility and suicide in relationship to (1) the wish to kill, (2) the wish to be killed, and (3) the wish to die. Menninger argued that each of these three wishes is present in every suicide, with one predominating in each.

Analytical Psychology

Jung (1959) and his followers have argued that suicide reflects an unconscious need for spiritual rebirth. As discussed by Wahl (1957), suicide represents a desire for renewal or resurrection to a different and better life. From this perspective suicide is seen as a magical and omnipotent act of regression toward rebirth of a new self. The following case of Billy illustrates well this type of thinking.

Case Example

Billy, a 12-year-old sixth grader, tried to hang himself in his bedroom closet but was discovered by his older brother. Recently humiliated at school by his peers, accused of being a "fag," Billy sought rebirth through suicide. When confronted by his parents after the attempt, Billy stated, "I know it sounds stupid, but I wanted a new life . . . I wanted to come back as a tough guy, someone no one would push around or call names."

Object Relations

Klein (1935) argued that suicide is a desperate intrapsychic act aimed at protecting internalized "good" objects from the death instinct and the destructive effects of one's internalized badness. Attachment to a rejecting object results in a split-off antilibidinal ego that internally reproduces the hostility of the rejecting object to libidinal needs. The libidinal ego is then hated and persecuted by the antilibidinal ego, which divides the ego against itself (Fairbairn, 1952; Guntrip, 1968).

Alternatively, Blanck and Blanck (1974) have argued that suicide reflects a wish to return to a state of symbiosis, resolving problems of separation and individuation. Therefore, suicide is a regressive act, a retreat to an early and safe symbiotic state where narcissistic equilibrium is reestablished. Issues related to symbiosis, dependency, and separation within a therapeutic relationship are central to the following case of Janet.

Case Example

Janet, a bulimic 16-year-old high school sophomore, took an overdose of her mother's sleeping pills. After being released from the emergency room to the care of her outpatient therapist, Janet said that she took the overdose because she was obsessed with the fear that her psychotherapist would leave her. Janet admitted to her doctor, "I thought it would be better to 'not-be' . . . and leave you before you get the chance to leave me . . . all alone."

Self-Psychology

Generally, proponents of self-psychology argue that psychopathology and its symptoms arise from fragmentation in the self structure (Kohut

& Wolf, 1978). Self fragmentation is reflected in lessened cohesion, more permeable boundaries, diminished energy and vitality, and a lack of internal balance. The experience of a crumbling self can be so painful that it must be avoided at all costs (e.g., through suicide). Alternatively, Baumeister (1990) conceptualizes suicide as an escape from aversive and painful self-awareness secondary to falling short of one's standards and expectations, which are internalized as failures. Shreve and Kunkel (1991), from a self-psychology/developmental perspective, assert that adolescent suicidal thoughts and behaviors are best understood as efforts to cope with *shame* and to communicate an intolerable sense of loss and lack of self-cohesion. A deteriorating sense of self, intense shame, and escape from unacceptable failure are central components to the suicide attempt of Jim in the following case.

Case Example

Jim, an 18-year-old high school senior all-state football star, miraculously survived a serious attempt to kill himself by crashing his car into a tree. As he was a popular senior, president of his class, and an A student, Jim's parents, friends, and school faculty were shocked by his behavior. Jim explained that his world had crumbled after he had injured his knee playing basketball, received a rejection to his Harvard application, and got a C on one of his exams.

Family Systems Theory

Another important line of theorizing arises from the family systems perspective (Minuchin, 1974). As discussed by Richman (1984, 1986), the essence of this approach is that disturbances in the family structure, including role conflicts and blurring of role boundaries, secretiveness and failures of communication, and rigidity with inability to accept change or tolerate crisis, have been thought to promote suicidal acting out within the family system. Also implicated is the potential influence of parental psychopathology and the influence of conscious and unconscious wishes by the parent to "kill off" the "expendable child," which may lead to the child's suicidal acting out. (See Sabbath, 1969; Shapiro & Freedman, 1987; Weissman, Paykel, & Klerman, 1972.) As a classic example, Kevin's suicide attempt can be understood at least partially in relation to family system dynamics.

Case Example

Kevin, a 13-year-old seventh grader, jumped out his second-story bedroom window after an intense fight with his manic-depressive mother. After being caught shoplifting, Kevin's mother had berated him and called him "a total pain in the ass." For many years Kevin's mother had blamed him for causing his father's drinking and abusiveness. She further claimed that Kevin was responsible for causing his older sister to run away from home.

Other Approaches

Maltsberger (1986) argues that to understand suicide vulnerability, one must grasp the two parts of the psychology of despair. First, the suicidal person experiences an absolutely intolerable affective state so painful that it cannot be endured. Second, the suicidal person recognizes the condition and gives up, abandoning the self as hopeless and unworthy of further concern. Suicidal people often have not developed their internal resources to self-soothe and must therefore rely solely on external resources for comfort. In such cases when external resources are absent, there is a profound sense of aloneness that puts ongoing survival in danger.

Smith (1985) has argued that psychoanalytic approaches to suicide have overemphasized the importance of single motivational phenomena, whether the unitary principle is that of loss, the death instinct, or separation-individuation. His ego vulnerability approach to suicide addresses intrapsychic mechanisms within a context of a particular pattern of ego organization. Central to this approach is the assumption that a matrix of dynamics and ego organization makes an individual vulnerable to suicidal crises. Thus, for a suicide to occur there must be a special loss of an unconscious life-guiding abstraction (one's "life fantasy" of internalized views of self and others) and a rigid, inflexible, vulnerable ego that chooses the denial of death as means of gaining intrapsychic control. The following case of Cindy clearly depicts her devastating loss of a guiding life fantasy.

Case Example

Cindy, a 17-year-old high school dropout, survived a serious overdose attempt after her mother discovered her unconscious in bed. A suicide note found on her desk spoke to her devastation over her breakup with her boyfriend who had just left to join the military. She had hoped they would marry and that she could live with him at his base. The final line in her note read "I quit, I can't take it any more, without Tom there's no reason to live . . . I would have been the best wife and mother . . . without him I'm alone . . . I have nothing."

Developmental Theory

As a closing theoretical consideration, each of the preceding approaches should be considered in relation to developmental theory. Clearly, adolescent suicidal behaviors occur within a critical developmental period where unique issues and needs are central. For example, adolescents are developmentally caught between two worlds: Needs for autonomy and independence paradoxically conflict with needs for dependency and a desire to remain a part of the family (Berman, 1984). As adolescents transition out of childhood, exploring and testing the world of adulthood, peer relationships and their influences become preeminent. Finally, many believe that adult identity is fundamentally established during adolescence (Erikson, 1968).

In truth, dynamically oriented thinkers have perhaps overemphasized, exaggerated, and even distorted the importance of adolescent development. Nevertheless, when clinically addressing adolescent suicidal behavior, it is virtually always useful to consider those developmental forces that make adolescence a unique stage of personal and interpersonal growth.

Case Example Continued

Referring back to Mark, a few of the previously discussed theoretical approaches apply. Mark certainly felt retroflex rage toward himself and his coach, and his potential suicide became a magical solution. In a single act of self-murder he could save himself while vengefully punishing his victimizer. Mark was an adolescent who had few friends and was largely disconnected from an inattentive and dysfunctional family system. His inherent ego vulnerability led him into a "friendship" that could help him escape his family. Yet this relationship created tremendous internal conflict and shame, which led to a fragmented sense of self and ultimately an unbearable level of despair.

EMPIRICAL CONSIDERATIONS

It is beyond the scope of this chapter to address comprehensively the relevant empirical data that has been obtained through various psychological autopsies studies. (See Brent et al., 1988; Shaffer & Gould, 1987; Shafii, Carrigan, Whittinghill, & Derrick, 1985.) Elsewhere, however, Berman and Jobes (1991) have summarized the major empirical findings within the research literature and presented overarching common themes of risk factors. The research themes most relevant to a dynamic understanding of adolescent suicide speak to (1) the importance of negative early life events, (2) disorders in psychological and characterological development, (3) the breakdown of intrapsychic defenses, (4) interpersonal isolation and alienation, and (5) negative views of self, others, and the future.

From a developmental research perspective, it is important to note that the recent studies of adolescence tend to contradict early and pervasive psychoanalytic theorizing of what is conventionally associated with the development of adolescents. Indeed, in contrast to Anna Freud's (1958) storm-and-stress model of adolescence where youth are plagued by anxiety, dread, and angst, recent data suggest that the vast majority of adolescents are *not* continuously in a state of misery, conflict, and suicidal angst. According to Offer (1987) and Abramowitz, Peterson, and Schulenberg (1984), the data indicate that most teens are well adjusted, get along with their parents and peers, adjust to social mores and values, and cope with their internal and external experience. However, these data do not suggest that the adolescent experience is by any means easy. Indeed, while most adolescents successfully navigate through this period, there is a distinct subgroup of adolescents at risk for suicide, who engage in deviant behaviors and have diagnosable psychopathology.

Case Example Continued

From an empirical standpoint, Mark, as a 19-year-old white male with access to a gun, matches the demographic profile of the modal adolescent completer. With regard to research themes, there is evidence of a painful and lonely childhood, a major depressive disorder, weakened ego defenses, interpersonal isolation, and an intolerably shameful and negative view of self.

PSYCHODYNAMIC CLINICAL INTERVENTION

Throughout the following discussion, the importance of the interactive and ongoing interplay between assessment and treatment is noted, and a distinction is made between clinical *management* of suicide risk and clinical *treatment* of the intrapsychic and interpersonal forces underlying suicide itself. Moreover, the importance of an initial assessment of risk, short-term and long-term treatment planning linked to initial and ongoing risk assessment, and clinical follow-through of the treatment plan must always be considered (Jobes & Berman, 1993).

Assessment of Suicide Risk

Maltsberger (1986, 1992) has provided perhaps the most comprehensive and contemporary psychodynamic contributions to the suicide risk assessment literature. His approach emphasizes an integrated formulation of clinical judgment—suicide risk assessment is an inductive, not intuitive, clinical activity. From the clinical plateau, the interviewing clinician must gather the raw information at hand, which includes (1) personal factors, (2) exterior factors, and (3) mental state phenomena.

Personal factors are epidemiological and clinical risk variables commonly associated with completed suicide (i.e., gender, race, age, psychopathology, access to lethal means). Other personal variables such as previous suicidal history, recent and significant losses, or a history of physical, sexual, and emotional abuse are included under this rubric.

Exterior factors include a range of external, environmental phenomena that affect the person in both immediate and long-term (characterological) ways. Maltsberger cites broad social and cultural influences (e.g., the cultural acceptance of guns), direct social influences (e.g., adolescent peer pressure), as well as family influences (e.g., the aforementioned effects of family conflict and psychopathology).

The final sector of raw information includes data obtained from the mental state examination. Central to this examination are details related to mental content (a suicide plan or death fantasy), cognition (constriction and disorders of thought), affect (self-hate, aloneness, murderous hate, hopelessness), intellectual functioning, and the patient's attitude toward the clinician (i.e., the quality of the therapeutic alliance).

This psychodynamic approach to the assessment of suicide risk therefore considers a synergy of personal, exterior, and mental state variables in relation to long-term characterological strengths and weaknesses, to determine the relative risk of suicide within a given patient. While only one contemporary psychodynamic perspective (emphasizing the clinical interview) has been presented here, alternative perspectives and the integrated use of interviews and psychological tests/scales to assess suicide risk can be found elsewhere (Bongar, 1991; Jobes, Eyman, & Yufit, 1990; Maris, Berman, Maltsberger, & Yufit, 1992).

Case Example Continued

Mark was assessed as possessing a moderately high level of risk in his initial outpatient interview. In terms of personal factors, Mark was a depressed white male who had access to guns and knew how to use them. Previous behaviors and conflictual love-hate feelings about his coach suggested the potential for future suicidal acting out. Considering exterior factors, Mark had only superficial peer relationships, and he came from a Southern, conservative, deeply religious family with contemptuous attitudes toward homosexuality. An evaluation of Mark's mental state revealed ongoing vague suicidal thoughts, cognitive constriction, a depressed and hopeless affect, and an uneasy (yet compliant) attitude toward the clinician. Characterologically, Mark was quite naive and immature, passive, and dependent.

Crisis Management

There is no particular "psychodynamic" approach to suicide crisis management per se since there is only one goal, which is distinctly atheoretical: The patient must remain physically safe and alive until the crisis situation has resolved. The aforementioned distinction between clinical *management* and *treatment* emphasizes the different roles and interventions required of the patient and therapist in the midst of crisis versus work conducted in ongoing treatment. Simply stated, there must be a living patient for treatment even to occur. Therefore, extraordinary means of maintaining safety and stability may be necessary. As discussed elsewhere (Berman & Jobes, 1991; Cimbolic & Jobes, 1990; Jobes & Berman, 1991), protection from self-harm may require the following steps: (1) Restricting access to means of death; (2) decreasing the patient's interpersonal isolation; (3) removing or decreasing agitation, anxiety, sleep loss; (4) structuring the treatment (e.g., increasing number of sessions); (5) working on problem-solving skills; (6) providing accessibility and availability to patient; (7) creating future linkages; (8) negotiating the maintenance of safety and the development of a contingency plan; and (9) effecting inpatient hospitalization in cases of clear and imminent suicide risk.

Case Example Continued

The initial treatment plan focused on maintaining Mark's safety. The gun his father had given him "for protection" at college was removed from his dorm room. Mark agreed to meet with his roommate and resident advisor to help increase his interpersonal support and decrease his isolation. Mark was continued on antidepressants, which his therapist gave him at their twice-weekly sessions. A carefully negotiated contingency plan for maintaining safety and making contact with the therapist (or another) was worked out. Most important, Mark agreed to resist his suicidal impulses to give therapy a chance.

Ongoing Treatment

Much has been written about crisis management. However, comparatively little has been written about the ongoing treatment of suicidal adolescents (from either a theoretical or an empirical perspective). Nevertheless, a number of psychodynamic treatment constructs may be quite useful in this regard.

The Therapeutic Alliance

Throughout the psychotherapy research literature, the quality of the therapeutic alliance is consistently cited as the most critical factor in successful psychotherapy (Goldfried, 1980), and there are a variety of methods for fostering the therapeutic alliance with adolescent patients (Berman & Jobes, 1991). Fundamentally, therapists must be capable of being a good-enough parent. Clinical management of the delicate balance between maintaining authority and being humanly accessible may be augmented by use of warmth within limits, appropriate self-disclosure, appropriate use of humor, and general flexibility (e.g., shorter or longer sessions depending on patient's tolerance). A collaborative and more active and directive approach often is useful. A clear understanding about confidentiality should be established, and the patient should be actively involved in treatment planning. The therapist's accessability and availability to the patient and criteria for considering hospitalization should be negotiated and understood as well.

Case Example Continued

Having long felt disconnected from others, as well as betrayed and violated by a trusted authority figure, the development of a strong therapeutic alliance was central to Mark's treatment. The alliance was therefore built around twice-weekly meetings (to provide object constancy), in which there was an emphasis on empathic listening, strategic use of self-disclosure, and a fair amount of humor (as Mark's life had become so grim). The therapeutic relationship itself was frequently discussed, and the therapist made efforts to be maximally flexible and responsive to Mark's expressed needs.

Transference

When working with suicidal adolescents, it is important to remember that a transferential dynamic often is already in place prior to the first contact. The clinician is generically seen as a member of the same generation from which the adolescent seeks autonomy, and a teen's associations to seeing a "doctor" or a "shrink" may have a long history that can be antagonistic to the kind of relationship needed for good treatment. In addition, the doctor's office may be a foreign (formal) place connoting certain labels, roles, and expectations, which the youth may strongly wish to avoid. Finally, as parents pay the bills and have legal rights related to treatment permission and clinical information, the underage patient may assume that the doctor will be on the parent's side.

Adolescent suicidal patients are often demanding and dependent, and may well replicate earlier disturbed relationships through transference. Therapists should accept and work through various projections and transferences, and strive to provide a potentially novel and stable good object relationship experience for the adolescent. Clinicians should give a clear and consistent message that they want to hear about, and can tolerate, the patient's painful affect. As Guntrip (1968) noted, basic "ego relatedness" is possible when the therapist shares in the patient's painful inner world as a *real* and good object.

Ideally, the clinician's major transferential role will be that of the good parent who does not expect behavior beyond the child's level of emotional maturity. Since teenagers typically struggle with issues of separation, helplessness, and dependency, these issues should be expected, accepted, and tolerated by the therapist. Critically, good parents (clinicians) nurture and gratify needs, but always within limits. Therefore, limit-setting is equally crucial to the patient, the therapist, and the overall efficacy of the psychotherapy.

Countertransference

Suicidal adolescents may regress and become increasingly demanding as dependency on the therapist evolves. Moreover, they may express anger and aggression as well as passivity—various behaviors that will test a therapist's patience and resolve and, perhaps, confirm the patient's own sense that he or she is undeserving of care or love.

Most therapists typically expect their patients to be motivated to utilize therapeutic help and actively engage in the process on their own behalf. Unfortunately, suicidal patients (particularly adolescents) generally do not fit the good patient role. Therapists confronted with such patients may respond with a variety of negative attitudes and feelings such as mild irritation, exasperation, wishes to be rid of the patient, even countertransferential hate (Maltsberger & Buie, 1974). If these attitudes and feelings are left unchecked, there may be iatrogenic effects via therapist withdrawal, malice, and avoidance.

To address countertransference, therapists should attempt to limit the number of seriously suicidal patients within their caseload to no more than a few at a time. It is also crucial that professional consultation be ready and available at all times. It is further helpful for therapists to keep abreast of institutional policies and procedures as well as relevant laws and statutes related to suicide and commitment procedures. Finally, self-monitoring and good record keeping are essential to bring to awareness unconscious negative thoughts and impulses that may interfere with effective psychotherapy.

Working-Through

Psychodynamic treatment of suicidality within the adolescent often requires a significant working-through period of intensive psychotherapy. This working-through phase may last from a few months to years depending on the degree of psychopathology. Other therapeutic modalities may be needed to supplement individual work. Family therapy, in particular, may prove to be a powerful adjunct to individual work (Brown, 1985; Richman, 1986). When appropriate, group therapy and psychopharmacotherapy should also be considered. (See Chapters 10 and 12.)

An integrated self-psychological and object relations approach can be quite valuable during the working-through period. Central to Kohut's self psychology is the concept of empathy—a process of gaining access to another's psychological state by "feeling oneself" into the other's experience (Wolf, 1988). In reference to transference phenomena, the self-psychology concept of "mirroring" (the therapist's acceptance and confirmation of the grandness, goodness, and wholeness of the patient's self) leads to important "selfobject" transferences. Through the "mirror transference," the patient may begin to experience universally felt narcissistic needs for another's recognition and appreciation of the self. As treatment progresses, another important selfobject transference, the "idealizing transference," may evolve as the patient's need for a calm, strong, wise, and good selfobject is met through the relationship with the therapist. Finally, alter-ego or "twinship transferences" are particularly powerful with adolescents in that they have intense affiliation needs to be alike and close to an important other.

Case Example Continued

In the case of Mark, use of empathic mirroring fostered a mirror transference such that he began to feel heard and appreciated by someone literally for the first time in his life. Fairly early in his treatment, idealizing and twinship tranferences began to emerge. A great deal of time was spent exploring these tranferences, which helped him gain perspective on his family relationships as well as his relationship with his coach. Mark's decision in his sophomore year to choose psychology as his undergraduate major had clear twinship-identification implications. The thorough exploration of this decision marked a significant turning point in his overall treatment.

The Therapeutic Relationship

From an object relations perspective, intrapsychic ego splitting can be healed through the therapeutic relationship. Guntrip (1968) describes the recovery process of psychotherapy in three stages. First, during rapport development, the patient needs a parent figure as a protector against intrapsychic pain and anxiety (i.e., a dependable rescuer from hopeless losing battles with problems the patient does not understand). The second stage, involving the development and analysis of transference, addresses how and why basic needs were (and are) not met in past (and present) relationships with the patient's actual parents and social network. Finally, in the third stage of regrowth/maturing, the patient begins to feel the impact of nonerotic stable parental love, which enables the child within to grow and possess its own individuality. In this final stage there is a maturing sense of selfhood that helps the patient to be separate without feeling cut off from key object relations.

Case Example Continued

Over time, Mark's transferential distortions of his therapist gave way to more reality-based perceptions. His perfect, all-knowing, all-powerful therapist came to be seen more as a real person, with strengths and weaknesses, who nevertheless genuinely cared for, respected, and appreciated Mark's specialness.

Under the umbrella of psychodynamically oriented psychotherapy, the common thread of healing centers on the importance of the therapeutic relationship. Within an appropriate, supportive, consistent, and caring relationship, the patient can grow through transference as well as the experience of the actual real relationship itself. Intrapsychic and interpersonal growth, which occur in relation to the therapist, enable internal suffering to be soothed and a fragmented self to become organized and cohesive. Where there is a cohesive self structure, internal and external sustaining resources, and good object relations, there is no need for suicide.

Termination

Berman and Jobes (1991) have argued that termination with the suicidal adolescent is perhaps better understood as a process of weaning. After long-term stabilization and sufficient therapeutic improvement, the once-suicidal adolescent can begin the process of separation. As treatment goals are attained, twice-a-week sessions may be reduced to once a week, which may be further reduced to twice monthly, monthly, quarterly, and so forth. It is suggested that the therapist remain a resource in the adolescent's life, such that contact can be made if needed. Contact can be maintained through infrequent postcards and "booster" sessions. These contacts serve to provide follow-up monitoring, a continued link, and/or the basis for a future referral.

Case Example Conclusion

In summary, Mark was seen in twice-weekly psychotherapy for three years and then weekly for one year. In terms of his initial suicide risk, it took about three months for him to become stabilized. As he immersed himself in his psychotherapy, his suicidal thoughts and impulses gradually faded away. As mentioned previously, the empathic mirroring and constancy of the supportive therapeutic relationship led to various selfobject transferences. As he worked through these transferences, Mark experienced sharp contrasts between the appropriate and empathically affirming intimacy of the therapeutic relationship and the inappropriate exploitive relationship with his coach. Over time, Mark was able to extricate himself from the hurtful relationship with his coach and develop age-appropriate peer relations. He came to see the relationship with the coach as more incestual than romantic. After graduation Mark's therapy came to a sensible end when he accepted a job in a neighboring state working in a group home for schizophrenics.

POTENTIAL PITFALLS

The potential pitfalls of a dynamic approach to treating suicidal adolescents can be avoided readily. Most potential psychodynamically based pitfalls arise when therapists rigidly follow an orthodox traditional drive-theory form of psychodynamic therapy. Clearly, what is not needed is an overly intellectual blank-screen, impersonal, or classically neutral therapist. Moreover, suicidal thoughts should never be interpreted blithely or dismissed as mere fantasy. Such thoughts must be taken very seriously and discussed as a potential reality. On another front, adolescence and suicidality both demand that the therapist take a more directive and active role in treatment, more than might be expected in some forms of dynamic therapy. Finally, an exclusive reliance on dynamically oriented individual psychotherapy is simply unwise since cognitive-behavioral work in problem-solving and skill building can be an especially effective treatment approach with suicidal adolescents (Berman & Jobes, 1991; Cimbolic & Jobes, 1990), and other interventions are quite often valuable (e.g., psychoactive medication and family therapy). While regressive historical dynamic work may be useful, adolescents need here-and-now skills for finding solutions to problems that arise in daily living.

CONCLUSION

A psychodynamic approach to the assessment, management, and treatment of suicidal adolescents can be quite effective and even life-saving. While no one theory or treatment strategy should ever be used exclusively, there is much within the psychoanalytic tradition to help guide one's clinical interventions. Perhaps most important, beyond crisis management, a psychodynamic approach to this clinical work holds the promise of actually treating (and resolving) the underlying causes of suicidality within the young person. When this occurs, the option of suicide becomes obsolete as new and better solutions to life's problems are possible.

REFERENCES

Abramowitz, R. H., Peterson, A. C., & Shulenberg, J. A. (1984). Changes in self-image during adolescence. In D. Offer, E. Ostrov, & K. I. Howard (Eds.), *Patterns of adolescent self-image* (pp. 19–28). San Francisco, CA: Jossey-Bass.

Baumeister, R. F. (1990). Suicide as escape from self. *Psychological Review, 97,* 90–113.

Berman, A. L. (1984, October). *The problem of teenage suicide.* Testimony presented before the U.S. Senate, Committee on the Judiciary, Subcommittee on Juvenile Justice, Washington, DC.

Berman, A. L., & Jobes, D. A. (1991). *Adolescent suicide: Assessment and intervention.* Washington, DC: American Psychological Association.

Blanck, G., & Blanck, R. (1974). *Ego psychology: Theory and practice.* New York: Columbia University Press.

Bongar, B. (1991). *The suicidal patient: Clinical and legal standards of care.* Washington, DC: American Psychological Association.

Brent, D. A., Perper, J., Goldstein, C., Kolko, D., Allan, M., Allman, C., & Zelenak, J. (1988). Risk factors for adolescent suicide: A comparison of adolescent suicide victims with suicidal inpatients. *Archives of General Psychiatry, 45,* 581–588.

Brown, S. (1985). Adolescents and family systems. In M. L. Peck, N. L. Farberow, & R. E. Litman (Eds.), *Youth suicide* (pp. 71–79). New York: Springer Publishing.

Cimbolic, P., & Jobes, D. A. (Eds.). (1990). *Youth suicide: Assessment, intervention, and issues.* Springfield, IL: Charles C. Thomas.

Erikson, E. (1968). *Identity: Youth in crisis.* New York: W. W. Norton.

Fairbairn, W. R. D. (1952). *Psychoanalytic Studies of the Personality.* London: Routledge and Kegan Paul.

Freud, A. (1958). Adolescence. *The Psychoanalitic Study of the Child, 13,* 261–277.

Freud, S. (1957). Mourning and melancholia. In J. Strachey (Ed. and Trans.), *The standard edition of the complete psychological works of Sigmund Freud* (Vol. 14, pp. 237–260). London: Hogarth Press. (Original work published 1917.)

Freud, S. (1955). Beyond the pleasure principle. In J. Strachey (Ed. and Trans.), *The standard edition of the complete psychological works of Sigmund Freud* (Vol. 18, pp. 3–66). London: Hogarth Press. (Original work published in 1920.)

Goldfried, M. R. (Ed.). (1980). Some views on effective principles of psychotherapy. *Cognitive Therapy and Research, 4,* 269–306.

Guntrip, H. (1968). *Schizoid phenomena, object relations and the self.* Madison, CT: International Universities Press.

Jobes, D. A., & Berman, A. L. (1991). Crisis intervention and brief treatment for suicidal youth. In A. Roberts (Ed.), *Contemporary perspectives on crisis intervention and prevention* (pp. 53–69). Englewood Cliffs, NJ: Prentice-Hall.

Jobes, D. A., & Berman, A. L. (1993). Suicide and malpractice liability: Assessing and revising policies, procedures, and practice in outpatient settings. *Professional Psychology: Research and Practice, 24,* 91–99.

Jobes, D. A., Eyman, J. R., & Yufit, R. I. (1990, April). *Suicide risk assessment survey.* Paper presented at the 23rd Annual Meeting of the American Association of Suicidology, New Orleans, LA.

Jung, C. G. (1959). The soul and death. In H. Feifel (Ed.), *The meaning of death* (pp. 3–15). New York: McGraw-Hill.

Klein, M. (1935). A contribution to the psychogenesis of manic-depressive states. *International Journal of Psycho-Analysis, 16,* 145–174.

Kohut, H., & Wolf, E. (1978). The disorders of the self and their treatment: An outline. *International Journal of Psycho-Analysis, 59,* 413–425.

Maltsberger, J. T. (1986). *Suicide risk: The formulation of clinical judgment.* New York: New York University Press.

Maltsberger, J. T. (1992). The psychodynamic formulation: An aid in assessing suicide risk. In R. Maris, A. L. Berman, J. T. Maltsberger, & R. I. Yufit (Eds.), *Assessment and prediction of suicide* (pp. 25–49). New York: The Guilford Press.

Maltsberger, J. T., & Buie, D. H. (1974). Countertransference hate in the treatment of suicidal patients. *Archives of General Psychiatry, 30,* 625–633.

Maris, R., Berman, A. L., Maltsberger, J. T., & Yufit, R. I. (Eds.). (1992). *Assessment and prediction of suicide.* New York: The Guilford Press.

Menninger, K. (1938). *Man against himself.* New York: Harcourt Brace.

Minuchin, S. (1974). *Families and family therapy.* Cambridge, MA: Harvard University Press.

Offer, D. (1987). In defense of adolescence. *Journal of the American Medical Association, 257,* 3407–3408.

Richman, J. (1984). The family therapy of suicidal adolescents: Promises and pitfalls. In H. S. Sudak, A. B. Ford, & N. B. Rushford (Eds.), *Suicide in the young* (pp. 393–406). Boston, MA: John Wright Publishing, Inc.

Richman, J. (1986). *Family therapy for suicidal people.* New York: Springer.

Sabbath, J. C. (1969). The suicidal adolescent—the expendable child. *Journal of American Academy of Child Psychiatry, 8,* 272–289.

Shaffer, D., & Gould, M. (1987). *A study of completed and attempted suicide in adolescents* (Progress report, Grant No. MH 38198). Rockville, MD: National Institute of Mental Health.

Shafii, M., Carrigan, S., Whittinghill, J. R., & Derrick, A. (1985). Psychological autopsy of completed suicide in children and adolescents. *American Journal of Psychiatry, 142,* 1061–1064.

Shapiro, E. R., & Freedman, J. (1987). Family dynamics of adolescent suicide. *Adolescent Psychiatry, 14,* 271–290.

Shneidman, E. S. (1980). Suicide. In E. S. Shneidman (Ed.), *Death: Current perspectives* (pp. 416–434). Palo Alto, CA: Mayfield Publishing Company.

Shreve, B. W., & Kunkel, M. A. (1991). Self-psychology, shame, and adolescent suicide: Theoretical and practical considerations. *Journal of Counseling and Development, 69,* 305–311.

Smith, K. (1985). An ego vulnerabilities approach to suicide assessment. *The Bulletin of the Menninger Clinic, 49,* 489–499.

Wahl, C. W. (1957). Suicide as a magical act. In E. S. Shneidman & N. L. Farberow (Eds.), *Clues to suicide* (pp. 22–30). New York: McGraw-Hill.

Weissman, M. M., Paykel, E. S., & Klerman, G. L. (1972). The depressed woman as a mother. *Social Psychiatry, 7,* 89–108.

Wolf, E. S. (1988). *Treating the self.* New York: The Guilford Press.

8

Cognitive Behavior Therapy of Adolescent Suicide Attempters

PAUL D. TRAUTMAN

Cognitive behavior therapy is a time-limited, problem-focused treatment that seeks to identify and change dysfunctional beliefs and behaviors. The treatment focuses on the *here and now*—the current individual and family situation—rather than on past experiences. The model presented in this chapter is derived from that of Beck, Rush, Shaw, and Emery (1979), which was developed for the treatment of depression in adults and has since been extended to the treatment of phobias, panic disorder, and anxiety disorders. Beck suggested that the depressed person has negative beliefs (dysfunctional thoughts) about him/herself, the world, and the future (the "cognitive triad" of depression), that these beliefs could be readily identified and modified, and that by so doing, the patient's mood and adaptive behavior would improve.

Trautman and Rotheram-Borus (1988) argued that it is difficult to believe that dysfunctional beliefs are primary and mood and behavior secondary; rather, mood, thoughts, and behavior are interactive, each impacting on the other. It follows that every problem may be conceptualized as having dysfunctional mood, thought, and behavioral components, and that problem-solving can begin by identifying and modifying any one component. In practice, with children and adolescents it is often easiest to start with modification of behavior. Behaviors are easier to observe and monitor than thoughts or mood. We first build behavioral success and later examine the child's beliefs and feelings about problem situations.

A suicide attempt, or the threat of one, is foremost a behavior, a behavior selected to solve interpersonal problems, relieve intense unpleasant mood, and resolve a contradictory and often fascinating set of dysfunctional beliefs. The therapist must first deal with this behavior to prevent its occurrence or recurrence. Is the patient to be hospitalized or to go home? The only absolute reasons for hospitalization are ongoing suicidal intent, psychosis, or lack of parental supervision. If discharge home is possible, what can the adolescent and his or her family *do* when suicidal thoughts recur, which they surely will? The patient needs to leave the office with a written plan—a list of people he or she can talk to or call, identified family members who will supervise and remove weapons and pills from the house, and a contract, sealed with a handshake, for no further suicidal behavior until the next appointment. This plan should be formulated with parental participation and assent.

CHARACTERISTICS OF THE COGNITIVE-BEHAVIORAL THERAPEUTIC RELATIONSHIP

These arrangements begin the cognitive-behavioral therapeutic relationship, which is characterized by collaboration between therapist and family, shared responsibility for the success of treatment, a therapeutic agenda for each session, written problem-solving tasks, homework assignments, and strategic planning for future difficulties. Cognitive behavior therapy with children and adolescents has another essential goal: increasing idealistically positive thoughts, feelings, and actions. The patient and family should not leave the first session without developing a list of their strengths—the things that *aren't* wrong. Suicidal patients are prone to engage in absolutist, all-or-nothing thinking (Beck et al., 1979, p. 194)—for example, "Nothing I do is right," "We'll never learn to get along." A list of strengths gives a message that "it's not all bad," counters a tendency (in therapists as well as families) to dwell on the negative and pathological, provides a social reward ("You did a good job"), forces the family to engage in a behavior—positive talk—incompatible with negativistic thinking, and begins to identify approaches to problem-solving consonant with the family's style.

Case Example

Elvira and her mother often quarreled, yet said they loved and were concerned about one another. The therapist had them list the ways they showed love and concern and had them practice these at home. This decreased the frequency and intensity of quarrels.

For a further discussion of positivity, see Trautman and Rotheram-Borus (1988).

Homework

The family is given homework assignments to do following each session. Homework assignments should build on skills learned during the session. They may be individual or family tasks and should be specific and targeted to the problem-solving needs of the family.

Case Example

Recovering in the intensive care unit from an overdose of digoxin, Jeanette prepared a list of "people I can call and things I can do when I'm upset" on a three-by-five-inch card. She was instructed to review this list every time she went to the bathroom. (She had secretly taken the overdose in the bathroom at home while her best friend sat in the living room.) Mother, who was working at the time of the overdose, complained that Jeanette had never spoken directly to her about what happened the afternoon of her overdose. Mother and daughter agreed to sit down together before the follow-up outpatient visit to review the events in detail; this homework assignment was chosen to test the capacity for, and to increase, mother-daughter communication.

Other typical homework assignments include:

1. "Caring days"—doing special favors and chores for a family member one day during the week.
2. Practicing communication skills such as eye contact, "I" statements, clear requests, feeling statements, stating how the other person feels (to develop understanding and empathy).
3. Sharing pleasant activities, such as window shopping, going to the park or to a movie, playing cards, cooking together, sharing meals (making sure the television is off).
4. Giving compliments.
5. Family meetings to air differences, plan activities, budgets, and so on.

6. Behavior chart of activities, chores, prosocial behaviors, homework, and the like.

7. Charting mood and activity.

8. Recording automatic and alternative thoughts and alternative behaviors.

Homework assignments continue the treatment process between office visits and reinforce the notion that the family can develop new skills to handle ongoing and new stressors. The assignments should be brief. Ask the family members if they will have time to do the task(s). Homework should be reviewed at the beginning of the next session. When and where did it happen? How did it go? Who said what? What difficulties were encountered? Homework helps the family and therapist evaluate the achievement of desired goals or the need for more focus on particular problems.

It's not unusual for homework not to be done, especially if written work was assigned, but most people will have at least thought about their homework and can do it at the beginning of the session. The therapist may need to help the family identify problems or negative assumptions (e.g., "Nothing will help us change, so why try?") that interfere with homework performance. (See Beck et al. [1979, pp. 56–57 and 408] for other reasons for not doing homework.)

Duration of Treatment and Frequency of Sessions

Adolescent suicide attempters differ greatly in the extent and severity of their problems, from acute crisis situations typical of younger adolescents (especially girls) to chronic, multiple individual and family problems encountered in older adolescents (especially boys). Cognitive therapy of adult depression and anxiety disorders typically lasts 20 to 30 sessions. However, in a pilot study of cognitive behavior therapy with adolescent suicide attempters, my colleague Mary Jane Rotheram-Borus, Ph.D., and I found that 15 sessions were often too many. In a more recent study (Trautman, Sanchez-Lacay, & Lewin, 1991), five sessions seemed adequate for girls, but at home follow-up we felt that families weren't using skills they had learned. This suggested to us that booster sessions at one- to two-month intervals might be helpful for maintaining treatment gains. Usually once-weekly sessions are scheduled, though twice-weekly sessions can be useful early in treatment for less stable patients. As the patient improves, frequency of sessions can be tapered down, say 2, 4, 7, 10, 14, and 22 weeks after the last weekly session—to ease the transition out of therapy and "boost" treatment gains. The value of telephone contact cannot be underestimated. (See Wasson, Gaudette, Whaley, Sauvigne, Baribeau, & Welch, 1992; Welu, 1977; and Chapter 13 in this volume.)

THE TREATMENT PROCESS

An advantage of cognitive behavior therapy is that it is systematic and therefore easy to learn and easy to teach. Being good at any therapy requires sound judgment, practice, and creativity; only the first of these is required to begin doing cognitive behavior therapy, plus a plan for the first two sessions. Each session begins by establishing an agenda, which typically includes: review of the previous session, review of homework, new work, new issues that the patient wants to discuss, selecting homework, review of what has been accomplished, and goals of next session.

The *goals* of cognitive behavior treatment with adolescent suicide attempters include:

1. Eliminate future suicide attempts.
2. Improve the adolescent's skills.
   a. Increase awareness of own feelings, thoughts, and actions.
   b. Increase ability to control feelings, thoughts, and actions.
   c. Increase frequency of pleasant and rewarding thoughts, feelings, and activities.
   d. Increase intra- and interpersonal problem-solving ability.
3. Improve family skills and relationships.
   a. Decrease parent-child conflict and increase shared activities.
   b. Increase parental tolerance of "normal" adolescent behavior and attitudes, and educate family about precipitants of suicidal behavior.
   c. Decrease criticism of the adolescent; increase praise, acknowledge strengths, communicate rules and goals clearly, share positive as well as negative feelings.
   d. Teach family problem-solving skills.

BRIEF OUTPATIENT THERAPY

What follows is an outline for a very brief outpatient therapy of approximately six to ten sessions in length. It is assumed that the patient is not actively suicidal, is nonpsychotic, and has a parent or caregiver who is willing to participate in treatment. Medications can be used concurrently without interference with the treatment process. I have become slower to prescribe antidepressants to the 25 percent of adolescent suicide attempters who meet criteria for major depressive disorder, having found that most patients' depressive symptoms resolve within a month's time (Trautman, Rotheram-Borus, Dopkins, & Lewin, 1991).

Session 1: Problems and Strengths; Positivity; Contract for No Suicidal Behavior; Treatment Contract

The family is seen together. The circumstances of the suicide attempt are reviewed briefly. Lists are prepared of the patient's and family's problems and strengths. These may be identified by patient, parents, therapist, or others. The suicide attempt or threat is problem number one. List every problem, however small, and make these specific, not global. For example, "Johnny is lazy" is too general; it is better to write "Johnny leaves his school bag on the sofa, he doesn't put his clothes in the hamper, there are pizza crusts and gum wrappers under his bed, he starts his homework at 10 P.M.," and so on. Try to make the list of strengths at least as long as the problem list, suggesting strengths if the family has difficulty coming up with them. Give a copy of the lists to the family to take home, and keep a copy for later use.

The lists of problems and strengths have immediate and future value. They concretize and delimit the scope of the problems, they let the family see that it's not all bad (this is often a great relief to the adolescent), they define the work of subsequent sessions (though problems always can be added later), they counteract the family's tendency to think negatively and globally, and they help trivialize some problems. It's hard to imagine a cure for laziness, but the pizza crust problem can be solved today!

A list of strengths also provides a shift from the negative—the problems that got the child into the clinic or office—to the positive. Early sessions should direct the family's attention to their strengths and their regard for one another, which they often have difficulty showing. Giving compliments is a useful exercise.

For example:

Therapist: Now, we don't just talk about problems in this office. It's important to talk about good things too, and giving compliments is a way to show you notice good things in people you care about. I like your shirt, Connie. That's a compliment. Now give me one.

Connie: What?!

Therapist: Do you like my tie?

Connie: Well . . .

Therapist: That's okay. This is just an exercise. Lie a little. Tell me you like my tie.

Connie: Nice tie.

Therapist: That's it. Now say it with enthusiasm, "Nice tie!"

Connie: Nice tie, Dr. T.!

Therapist: Right! Now it's Mom's turn to give you a compliment.

Mom: She keeps her room nice.

Therapist: Good. Only tell her, not me.

Mom: I'm proud of the way you keep your room.

Connie: Thank you.

Therapist: Excellent. I forgot to say "thank you" before. It's very important to acknowledge a compliment; otherwise, people tend to stop giving them.

In this, as in other exercises, the therapist models and shapes the behavior he or she seeks to teach, praising any effort while maintaining a tone of enthusiasm and hopefulness. The therapist should use his or her own and the family's sense of humor, including a little teasing and self-deprecation, without being insincere, insensitive to other's distress, or hostile.

The first session concludes with a contract for no further suicidal behavior and a homework assignment. I like the patient to look me in the eye and say, "I don't feel suicidal now and I won't do anything to hurt myself between now and next Tuesday, when I have my next appointment." A list of people to call and things to do is prepared, in case he or she does feel suicidal again. The homework assignment should reinforce a skill practiced during the session. For example, the family might have a brief meeting on Friday night to: (1) give a compliment to each family member and receive one, and (2) plan a mutually enjoyable family activity for a weekend day. Rules for meeting include: (1) no TV or telephone calls and (2) no criticism or arguing is allowed. (Arguing at other times is okay, and this should be so stated.)

Finally, the date and time of the next and all subsequent visits are agreed upon. Contracting for a small number of visits keeps the thera- pist and family on their toes. If important issues remain at the last ses- sion, further visits and booster sessions can be negotiated.

Session 2: Feeling Thermometer; Review of Homework and Compliments

Adolescents, particularly younger ones, often feel overwhelmed when problems arise, and have difficulty articulating their thoughts and feel- ings and formulating a solution. Before adolescents can identify their dysfunctional (automatic) thoughts, they need help identifying their moods and the intensity of those moods in a variety of situations. The Feeling Thermometer (Wolpe, 1958; also called the Subjective Units of Distress Scale, or SUDS) was adapted to facilitate identification and discussion of mood states (Trautman & Rotheram-Borus, 1988). The Feeling Thermometer is a single sheet of paper with a 100-point scale drawn down the left-hand margin. On this scale 100 (at the top) is "the worst you ever felt" and 0 is "the best—no problems whatsoever." The adolescent briefly describes situations that fit these extremes—often the precipitant of the suicide attempt is the worst—and the associated mood: for example, mad, sad, excited. Other examples, neither so bad nor so good, are filled in. "When Dad yelled at me for coming in late" might be rated 62 on one adolescent's chart but only 17 on another's. Problems from the problem list can be fit onto the scale. About five to seven examples will suffice to start; others will be added in later ses- sions. Arbitrarily, situations rated 30 or less are defined as "not so bad" and don't require much discussion. (However, one school-phobic adolescent rated his worst problem—going to school—a 30, so that we discussed many problems in the 10-to-30 range. Be flexible.)

Adolescents often have an "Aha!" experience with this exercise as they realize that not every bad thing that happens is the worst thing, and that there are many problem situations that they handle without much difficulty. Often they have difficulty finding examples in the middle range, tending to think of situations at the extremes, and the therapist may have to suggest examples from the problem list or men- tion situations with which other adolescents typically have difficulty. Each adolescent's Feeling Thermometer is unique, a kind of thumbnail sketch of his or her temperamental style and coping abilities. The goal of later sessions will be to find ways to lower the SUDS of "high-temperature" situations to a manageable level.

The Feeling Thermometer may be developed with or without the other family members present; in either case, they should be made familiar with the concept of identifying the strength of feelings. The adolescent may or may not be willing to show the scale to his or her parents. He or she should retain a copy, as should the therapist, for use in later sessions. Homework should be reviewed with the whole family. In addition to reviewing problems since the last session, ask "What went well?" Ask the adolescent in every session if he or she felt suicidal since the last visit, and if not, why not. "What did you do to take care of yourself?" A new homework assignment might be to practice compliments and to add further examples to the Feeling Thermometer.

Sessions 3 and 4: Thought and Action Sheet—Problem Situation, SUDS, Automatic Thoughts, Alternative Behaviors and Thoughts; "I" Statements

The goal of these sessions is to introduce a formal method of problem-solving: how to break down a problem into its component parts and to generate possible solutions. Bring out the Feeling Thermometer and briefly review the last session and homework. What examples were added? What is the adolescent's "temperature" right now? What is it when giving or receiving a compliment? What's his or her SUDS when Mom and Dad yell at each other? When family members are present in the session, ask their SUDS too.

The Thought and Action Sheet is now introduced. It was adapted from Beck and associates (1979) and consists of a single sheet of paper with headings for each of the components of a problem, separated by plenty of space for written responses:

Event (problem)
Feeling and SUDS
Automatic Thoughts
What did you do?
Goals (What would be a good outcome?)
Alternative Behaviors
Alternative Thoughts

Reassessment: Have the goals been met? (If not, test second-choice alternatives.)

Begin with any problem, either a new one that arose since the last session or one from the problem list. Some problems have obvious, easy solutions, and the family will get a quick sense of accomplishment by starting with one of these; other adolescents may prefer starting with the biggest or most pressing problem. For example:

Therapist: When your SUDS is high, when you're "hot," you'd like to cool off, and in this session and the next we're going to discuss a way of lowering your SUDS. First you have to identify the problem, describe it. Then ask yourself, "What's my SUDS? Can I handle it?" Let's begin with one of the problems on your problem list or with a new problem you had this week. Describe it briefly.

Once a problem has been described, along with associated affects and a SUDS score for each, explain what automatic thoughts are.

Therapist: When we're upset, we all tend to have "automatic thoughts." These are the things we say to ourself in the heat of the moment; they tend to be negative and absolute, like, "This is the worst thing that's ever happened" or "I hate that guy" or "I'm so stupid" or "I'll never be happy." Do you ever find yourself thinking that way? For example, what you were thinking when your mom told you to pack your bags?

Younger adolescents may need help putting their automatic thoughts into words. Often the therapist already will have heard several of the child's or parent's automatic thoughts and can repeat them, or can give examples that other adolescents have mentioned in similar situations. Automatic (dysfunctional) thoughts are further characterized by their tendency to occur repetitively and to be situation-specific, by their surface plausibility, and by their accessibility to consciousness (unlike "unconscious" thought, which by definition motivates behavior but is not readily accessible). The automatic thoughts characteristic of depression include a "cognitive triad"—a negative view of oneself, the world, and the future (Beck et al., 1979, p. 11; see also Burns, 1980, pp. 40–41, for a useful list of definitions of a variety of cognitive distortions).

The therapist must resist the temptation to refute these automatic distortions. Parents usually cannot resist, and may say, for example, "Of course you're not ugly! You're really very handsome and Aunt Emma says so every time she sees you." Rather, the goal of the cognitive therapist is to see the world as the patient sees it (this makes the patient's behavior logical) and then to help him or her examine the extent to which his or her assumptions are true. (See Sessions 7–9 that follow.) Thus it's helpful to say "So you believe you're ugly. Well, no wonder you avoid eye contact, and refuse to answer when your friends telephone. I would too. What else does feeling ugly make you do, or stop you from doing?"

The next steps on the Thought and Action Sheet are: (1) to simply state the goal (What would be a reasonable outcome for this problem?); and (2) to list as many possible solutions as the adolescent, family, and therapist can think of.

Case Example

Rhonda complained that her father yelled at her for talking too long on the phone with her boyfriend; she felt depressed (SUDS 60) and angry (SUDS 92). Her automatic thoughts were "I hate him. He's never nice to me." She yelled back, slammed the door, and was grounded. Her goal was to be able to talk on the phone whenever she wanted without being scolded.

Rhonda's alternative behavior list included: Yell back, threaten to kill myself, stay in my room, write in my diary, take another overdose, ask Mother to intervene, go to girlfriend's house, run away, refuse to let him kiss me, talk to him after he's calmed down, dump the boyfriend, and attend Alanon. Her alternative thoughts included: Say to myself "Keep cool, take a deep breath, it's not so bad, you can handle it," remember that he's irritable when he drinks but that sometimes he's nice, think about going away to college next year, picture him hanging him by his thumbs.

A good list of alternatives is a long list and one that includes good, bad, and impossible solutions. To promote a long list, participants should be free to suggest anything, without censoring. A long list counteracts the automatic thought "There's nothing I can do" and is an essential prerequisite of effective problem-solving (Spivack, Platt,

& Shure, 1976). Of course, family members also should understand the important distinction between *talking* about something and actually *doing* it. If someone in the family doesn't mention suicidal behavior as an option, the therapist should, for two reasons: (1) Families often avoid talking about "it," and (2) the adolescent will want to weigh the advantages and disadvantages of suicidal behavior. See further discussion of advantages and disadvantages in the next section.

As the therapist teaches the Thought and Action Sheet approach to problem dissection, he or she also should continue to work on improving family communication. Giving and receiving compliments was the first step; now "I" statements are introduced. These are simple direct statements about one's feelings and desires. For example: "I feel worried when you stay out after 10 P.M."; "I'm happy when you invite my friends over"; "I feel hurt when you don't listen when I'm speaking to you." Families of suicide attempters often fail to communicate directly in this way, avoid expression of positive and negative affect, leave things unspoken (e.g., avoiding confrontation or sulking), assume others can read one's mind ("He knows how I feel"), or make vague and indirect statements ("This place is a mess" rather than "I want you to put your coat and book bag in your room now, please").

Like other social skills, "I" statements need to be practiced in the session. The therapist models the skill, asks each family member to make an "I" statement, and provides feedback: "That was a nice, clear statement, but I noticed you didn't look her in the eye. Try it again, and just a little louder. That's it!" The person being spoken to should be told not to respond defensively or try to help the subject feel differently, but just to acknowledge having heard and to indicate that he or she understands how the subject feels. This begins the work of social perspective-taking—that is, knowing how others think and feel about a given situation—a skill in which children with externalizing disorders are particularly deficient (Kendall, Zupan, & Braswell, 1981; Lochman, White, & Wayland, 1991).

Homework might include asking the adolescent to complete a Thought and Action Sheet up to the point of alternatives and asking the family to practice "I" statements three times during the intervening week.

Sessions 5 and 6: Evaluating Pros and Cons; Testing Solutions; Practicing Social Skills Including Social Perspective-Taking and Assertiveness; Family Rules and Regulations

Begin by reviewing the newly completed Thought and Action Sheet, and ask the family members to repeat their "I" statements. In practice, many adolescents won't have actually written out their responses but will have thought about them. A brief discussion serves as a review of the skills covered in the last two sessions.

Every alternative behavior and thought has its advantages and disadvantages (pros and cons); if the latter outweigh the former, it's not a good solution and should be given up. Families are taught to list these, to narrow down the options, and to test out one or more solutions. Did it work? If not, why not? Try again, with modifications, or try something else.

Therapist: Let's talk about some of your alternative behaviors. When your father yells at you, you think of taking another overdose. What would be some of the advantages of that?

Rhonda: He'd be sorry. I'd get out of the house for a while. Maybe my mother would leave him.

Therapist: And disadvantages?

Rhonda: I might be dead! I'd have to drink that gross black stuff again. They'd probably both hit me. It would hurt my mother and I'm not mad at her. I'm not really mad at him now either; it seems silly.

Therapist: So on balance, what do you think?

Rhonda: No way!

Therapist: What about another alternative?

Rhonda: Well, if he's sober, sometimes he listens. Sometimes they let me talk on the phone, and sometimes they don't. Why don't they make up their minds?

Therapist: Any disadvantages to talking to him about it?

Rhonda: He's so stubborn. It's better if my mother's there.

Therapist: Why not try it right now? Tell him how you feel and what you want.

Skills need to be practiced in the session, with the therapist providing immediate feedback and shaping; for example, "That's good, that's not, is that what you really want to say? Can you say that again without sounding so angry? Try saying this, watch how I would do it." Role reversal can be very useful, with the daughter taking the father's part, the therapist the mother's, and so forth.

When the "problem person" is not present (a boyfriend or teacher, for example), the adolescent can take that role ("You're the expert on how he acts"), and a fairly specific dialogue can be rehearsed, including alternative responses, depending on how things go in vivo. The homework assignment would then be to have this conversation with the "problem person" and report on the results.

Finally, give family members an opportunity to suggest rules and regulations for the adolescent. This discussion began in the first visit with the no-suicide contract in which the family agreed about a tightly structured plan of close supervision and monitoring of suicidal ideation. Let this evolve into a more general discussion of rules and regulations. Parents of suicide attempters often are unclear about rules and inconsistent about enforcement. This leads to arguments and stretching of rules. Given the opportunity, adolescents can be surprisingly reasonable about the household chores and curfews they suggest for themselves. Encourage discussion and negotiation. Explore the automatic thoughts of rigid parents.

Sessions 7–9: Gathering Evidence; Evaluating Consequences; Self-Attributions

The later sessions of a brief cognitive behavior treatment are devoted to applying the problem-solving techniques previously learned to a variety of intra- and extrafamilial situations, particularly generating alternative behaviors and thoughts, weighing their advantages and disadvantages, trying out new solutions, and evaluating the outcome. Many adolescents need to acquire new skills (because of cognitive *deficits*) as well as to modify existing beliefs (because of cognitive *distortions*) (Kendall, 1985). For example, they may need to learn how to be assertive without being provocative or aggressive. Similarly, as anger is the chief affect associated with suicide attempts, particular attention may need to be devoted to anger control—when it is appropriate, when it is not, how to use it constructively, how to temper it, and so forth.

Much of what has been discussed until this point has to do with things the patient and family can do or say to solve problems. This is because, while change can occur by modification of thought, feeling, or action, often it is easiest to modify behavior first; that is, to think of something quick and easy to *do*. However, it does not follow that as people's behavior changes so their beliefs change; often there is a lag. Families frequently will come to a session and say, "We didn't do our homework, everyone's fighting, nothing has changed," when in fact they had a family meeting, mother and daughter went window shopping on Saturday, the children cleared the table without being asked, and only one major argument happened, as opposed to three the week before. The therapist needs to point out the changes—having the family keep behavioral charts is useful so that one can point to hard evidence—and to ask the family to develop an alternative belief (e.g., "We did have one argument, but we discussed it in the family meeting, and everyone has been cooperating better; we made some progress").

This technique of gathering evidence pro and con about an automatic thought ("Nothing has changed") is a useful approach to changing cognitions. If the adolescent says, "Nobody loves me, so I might as well be dead," the appropriate tack is "Maybe that's true, maybe it isn't, I don't know you well enough yet, let's gather some evidence. Let's list some things people did or said that made you believe they didn't love you. Then let's list some loving things. And are there other reasons for living, besides being loved?" The adolescent might need to gather further evidence at home, by taking a poll, for example, or by observing body language, eye contact, and voice tone. This is followed by an alternative statement that is a more objective summary of the facts.

Self-attributions are the interpretations one makes about good and bad events. The dysfunctional perception of negative events has been characterized by internal, stable, and global attributions (Abramson, Seligman, & Teasdale, 1978). For example, when something goes wrong, the adolescent may think, "It's my fault, everything I do is wrong, nothing will ever change." Similarly, positive events are dismissed as external, unpredictable, and isolated ("So what if I got an A? It was an easy test and I'm sure to fail all my finals"). Bad things happen that adolescents cannot control: Teachers have bad days and say unkind things, parents argue, boyfriends fall out of love. But adolescents *can* control how they talk to themselves about these events, isolating the negative and rewarding themselves for the positive. Every dysfunctional belief has a rational, reasonable alternative. For example:

> *Dysfunctional attribution:* "My mom and dad blamed one another because I failed math. I should never have been born."

> *Alternative attribution:* "They argue no matter what I do. They never take responsibility for their own faults. I can't change them. Maybe I can study with my friend Jill. She's good at math."

In-office and homework exercises can be developed that increase the adolescent's (and family's) ability to recognize automatic thoughts and counter them with coping self-instructional thinking ("Okay, stay calm, I can handle this. Now let's think what's the best way out of this mess?").

Session 10: Final Session—Review of Problems and Treatment; Outstanding Problems; Further Sessions? Booster Sessions?

As treatment progresses, the therapist routinely should remind the family of the number of sessions remaining in the treatment contract, so that all participants have an opportunity to bring their concerns to the agenda at some point. The treatment should be flexible enough to allow new issues to arise, but sufficiently structured so that no one comes to a sessions ignorant of what is to take place, and no session progresses without structure. This is why it is important to set an agenda at the beginning of each session. (See "The Treatment Process" earlier.)

The last meeting is devoted to a review of the entire treatment: What were the presenting problems? How were these addressed? What has the family learned? How comfortable are the parents with the adolescent's current adjustment? Are there any worries about suicidal behavior? What outstanding problems are there? Should we stop, or shall we establish new goals and a new time frame?

The value of "booster" sessions was mentioned previously. Many acute crises that precipitate suicide attempts quickly resolve as family members adopt their best behavior, only to reemerge as old habits revive. Follow-up sessions encourage the family to continue to use newly acquired skills and allow discussion of reemergent problems.

SUMMARY AND CONCLUSIONS

In this chapter a brief, problem-solving approach to individual and family work with the adolescent suicide attempter or ideator was outlined. The adolescent suicide attempter has acute problems that are rooted in chronic family dysfunction (de Wilde, Kienhorst, Diekstra, & Wolters, 1992; King, Raskin, Gdowski, Butkus, & Opipari, 1990; Trautman, 1989), so that individual and family therapy are invariably essential.

The cognitive-behavioral approach is a collaboration between therapist and family to identify problems, strengths, and solutions to here-and-now difficulties. The therapist must view the world as the patient views it in order to understand the patient's mood and behavior. He or she then suggests that alternative beliefs and actions are possible; these are listed and tested systematically. Mood and beliefs are subsequently reexamined: Am I coping better? Do I feel better? If not, test another alternative. Families readily adapt to the collaborative, problem-solving approach of cognitive therapy. The therapist wants to discharge the family with set of skills for solving future difficulties.

Finally, an effective cognitive-behavioral therapist is active, assertive, explanatory, and responsive (Dulcan, 1984; Kolvin et al., 1981; Ricks, 1974; Shaffer, 1984); he or she models interpersonal problem-solving skills (Meichenbaum & Goodman, 1971) and provides positive feedback (Trautman & Rotheram-Borus, 1988). The term "cognitive therapy" has always struck the writer as having a rather naive and cerebral ring to it ("Just alter your cognitions and you'll feel better"), whereas in practice, cognitive therapy with children and adolescents is logical, practical, vernacular, and fun.

REFERENCES

Abramson, L. Y., Seligman, M. E. P., & Teasdale, J. D. (1978). Learned helplessness in humans: Critique and reformulation. *Journal of Abnormal Psychology, 87,* 49–74.

Beck, A. T., Rush, A. J., Shaw, B. F., & Emery, G. (1979). *Cognitive therapy of depression.* New York: The Guilford Press.

Burns, D. D. (1980). *Feeling good: The new mood therapy.* New York: New American Library.

de Wilde, E. J., Kienhorst, I. C. W. M., Diekstra, R. F. W., & Wolters, W. H. G. (1992). The relationship between adolescent suicidal behavior and life events in childhood and adolescence. *American Journal of Psychiatry, 149,* 45–51.

Dulcan, M. K. (1984). Brief psychotherapy with children and their families: The state of the art. *Journal of the American Academy of Child Psychiatry, 23,* 544–551.

Kendall, P. C. (1985). Toward a cognitive behavioral model of child psychopathology and a critique of related interventions. *Journal of Abnormal Child Psychology, 13,* 357–371.

Kendall, P. C., Zupan, B. A., & Braswell, L. (1981). Self-control in children: Further analyses of the Self-Control Rating Scale. *Behavior Therapy, 12,* 667–681.

King, C. A., Raskin, A., Gdowski, C. L., Butkus, M., & Opipari, L. (1990). Psychosocial factors associated with urban adolescent female suicide attempters. *Journal of the American Academy of Child and Adolescent Psychiatry, 29,* 289–294.

Kolvin, E., Garside, R. F., Nicol, A. R., Macmillan, A., Wolstenholme, F., & Letch, I. M. (1981). *Help starts here: The maladjusted child in the ordinary school.* London: Tavistock.

Lochman, J. E., White, K. J., & Wayland, K. K. (1991). Cognitive-behavioral assessment and treatment with aggressive children. In P. C. Kendall (Ed.), *Child and adolescent therapy, cognitive-behavioral procedures* (pp. 25–65). New York: The Guilford Press.

Meichenbaum, D., & Goodman, J. (1971). Training impulsive children to talk to themselves: A means of developing self-control. *Journal of Abnormal Psychology, 77,* 114–126.

Ricks, D. F. (1974). Supershrink: Methods of a therapist judged successful on the basis of adult outcomes of adolescent patient. In D. F. Ricks, A. Thomas, & M. Roff (Eds.), *Life history research in psychopathology* (vol. 3, pp. 275–297). Minneapolis: University of Minnesota Press.

Shaffer, D. (1984). Notes on psychotherapy research among children and adolescents. *Journal of the American Academy of Child Psychiatry, 23,* 552–561.

Spivack, G., Platt, J., & Shure, M. (1976). *The problem-solving approach to adjustment.* San Francisco, CA: Jossey-Bass.

Trautman, P. D. (1989). Specific treatment modalities for adolescent suicide attempters. In Alcohol, Drug Abuse, and Mental Health Administration, *Report of the Secretary's Task Force on Youth Suicide (vol. 3): Prevention and interventions in youth suicide* (pp. 253–263) (DHHS Publication #[ADM]89-1623). Washington, DC: Superintendent of Documents, United States Government Printing Office.

Trautman, P., & Rotheram-Borus, M. J. (1988). Cognitive behavior therapy with children and adolescents. In A. J. Frances & R. E. Hales (Eds.), *American Psychiatric Press review of psychiatry* (vol. 7, pp. 584–607). Washington, DC: American Psychiatric Press.

Trautman, P. D., Rotheram-Borus, M. J., Dopkins, S., & Lewin, N. (1991). Psychiatric diagnoses in minority female adolescent suicide attempters. *Journal of the American Academy of Child and Adolescent Psychiatry, 30*, 617–622.

Trautman, P. D., Sanchez-Lacay, A., & Lewin, N. (1991, May). *Brief treatment of adolescent suicide attempters*. Paper presented at the 144th Annual Meeting of the American Psychiatric Association, New Orleans, LA.

Wasson, J., Gaudette, C., Whaley, F., Sauvigne, A., Baribeau, P., & Welch, H. G. (1992). Telephone care as a substitute for routine clinic follow-up. *Journal of the American Medical Association, 267*, 1788–1793.

Welu, T. C. (1977). A follow-up program for suicide attempters: Evaluation of effectiveness. *Suicide and Life Threatening Behavior, 7*, 17–30.

Wolpe, J. (1958). *Reciprocal inhibition therapy*. Palo Alto, CA: Stanford University Press.

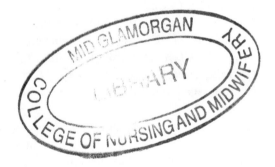

9

Being the Family's Therapist
An Integrative Approach

JAMES K. ZIMMERMAN AND
VALERIE A. LA SORSA

In the past 15 years, there has been a powerful movement toward integrating approaches to psychotherapy on the levels of both theoretical constructs and technical interventions (Arkowitz, 1991; Beitman, Goldfried, & Norcross, 1989; Lazarus & Messer, 1991; Norcross & Grencavage, 1989). One area in which integration has been particularly active is in the combination of individual and family treatment (Carter, 1987; Case & Robinson, 1990; Guerney & Guerney, 1987; Kaslow & Racusin, 1990; Turgay, 1989). Although there are those who continue to debate the wisdom of this movement (Haley, 1987; Nichols, 1987), there is a growing body of literature suggesting that psychotherapy integration is becoming acceptable and respected by a wide range of clinicians from various schools of thought (Beitman et al., 1989; Feldman, 1985; Karasu, 1979; Pinsof, 1983; Wachtel, 1991). For example, Karasu (1979) concludes that "instead of a partisan allegiance to, and utilization of, a single system to the rejection of all others, more than one therapy or parts of many therapies may be combined in producing the most potent therapeutic regimes" (p. 562). In another instance, Beitman, Goldfried, and Norcross (1989) assert that clinicians have begun to recognize the "inadequacies of any one system and the potential value of others" (p. 138).

Definitions of "Integration"

One confusing and unresolved issue in the integrative treatment literature is the exact definition of the term "integration" and on what levels of conceptualization this process occurs in a given therapist's practice (Beitman et al., 1989; Case & Robinson, 1990). Three modes

174

of integration—technical eclecticism, common factorism, and theoretical integration—have been delineated (Arkowitz, 1991; Norcross & Grencavage, 1989), although debate continues as to which mode is the most appropriate (Lazarus & Messer, 1991). For example, Lazarus argues that integration should occur on the level of technical eclecticism (i.e., the employment of the most effective techniques without concern for the theories that spawned them), while Messer suggests that attempts to do so ignore the fact that techniques are infused with constructs of the theory from which they were derived, and that integration on the theoretical level is therefore most appropriate (Lazarus & Messer, 1991). Elsewhere, Turgay (1989) suggests that integration must occur through bringing together the "integratable parts" of well-recognized theoretical and therapeutic approaches, while also considering the integration of target systems for intervention (e.g., individual, family, school, etc.).

In this chapter we will present and discuss a model for integrating different treatment modalities and theoretical positions in interventions with suicidal adolescents and their families in a brief treatment context. Our approach is most consonant with that of Turgay (1989), in that we attempt to interweave "integratable parts" theoretically, technically, and with regard to the target system for intervention. With respect to modalities, individual and family approaches are integrated, while in some cases including couples' sessions with the adolescent's parents. Regarding theoretical integration, the approach draws upon family systems, psychodynamic, and developmental perspectives.

Integration of Modalities of Treatment

There is strong justification in the literature for bridging individual and family perspectives in treating suicidal adolescents. Wachtel and Wachtel (1986) maintain that "neither the dynamics of individuals or the context in which they operate can be ignored, and that the two codetermine each other in ways that it is essential to understand" (p. 2). With respect to the treatment of children and adolescents, other authors repeatedly cite the need to integrate theoretical perspectives, in order to understand the complexity of individual behavior and family functioning (Feldman & Powell, 1992; Kirschner & Kirschner, 1986; Wachtel & Wachtel, 1986) and to end the limiting effects of exclusivity in theoretical conceptualization (Nichols, 1987). Levant and Haffey (1981) maintain that "the child needs to be seen within the context of his/her family, yet the child (as well as the parents) exists not only as a member of the family system, but also as an individual at a certain stage of development in his/her life cycle" (p. 139).

Technical Integration

In the technical realm, a fluid approach most suits the needs of the cases to be described in this chapter. This approach integrates modalities, is dictated by the issues that arise during the course of treatment, and is implemented by a single therapist. Early in the literature on treatment integration, Kaffman (1965) and Charny (1966) separately advocated such a flexible treatment approach to meet the diverse needs of families and individuals. Charny proposed "a psychotherapy where individual and family interviews are utilized concurrently in a flexible, unfolding sequence that grows out of the flow or movement of each particular case" (1966, p. 179).

In the remainder of this chapter, we outline how this approach functions in our work. Initially, we describe the clinical context in which this treatment approach has evolved. Following that, we present some of the fundamental dynamics that we see as central to the experience of suicidal adolescents and their families, illustrating with case materials the ways in which this understanding influences our psychotherapeutic stance. Finally, we discuss some relevant technical issues that arise in the context of the approach to treatment which we advocate.

THE CLINIC

The Adolescent Depression and Suicide Program (ADSP) at Montefiore Medical Center/Albert Einstein College of Medicine, Bronx, New York, is a brief treatment, outpatient clinic designed to provide mental health services for suicidal adolescents and their families. The population largely derives from underprivileged, minority, inner-city backgrounds; many of the families have only one biological parent in the household, most often the mother, and acrimonious relationships between the biological parents are common. Typically, adolescents are referred to the clinic soon after they have made a suicide attempt.

The clinic provides crisis intervention, extensive evaluation, and time-limited psychotherapy to these adolescents and their families. Because the stay in treatment is limited to approximately three months, there is strong pressure to accomplish as much as possible in a short period of time. As a result, there has been a concerted effort to develop and implement treatments for this population that can exert powerful therapeutic leverage quickly.

It is within this crucible, then, that our approach to treatment has been formed, and we have found that the most effective stance is to position ourselves as the "family's therapist." Our intent is to be of service to the family system either as a whole or in various constituent parts, much as a trusted family doctor treats each and all members of a family (Kirschner & Kirschner, 1990; Vane & DeMaria, 1988). In this way, we are able to gain direct access quickly not only to the systems issues at hand but also to salient individual and subsystem (e.g., couples) issues.

FUNDAMENTAL DYNAMICS

In recent years a substantial body of literature has related suicidality in adolescents to family issues. Research has shown that family problems are frequently considered a major precipitant in suicide attempts among adolescents (Pfeffer, 1989; Spirito, Brown, Overholser, & Fritz, 1989; Tishler, McKenry, & Morgan, 1981). Specifically, family disruptions, including losses (through divorce, absence, and death) and physical and sexual abuse, have been found to relate to attempted and completed suicide (Landau-Stanton & Stanton, 1985; Pfeffer, 1989; Shaffer, 1974; Shafii, Carrigan, Whittinghill, & Derrick, 1985; Spirito et al., 1989).

It is thus apparent that the behavior of adolescent suicide attempters quite often is strongly influenced by family dynamics. Conversely, a suicide attempt by an adolescent also has a powerful impact on the development of his or her family system. It follows logically, then, that a combined focus on family systems issues, individual dynamics, and developmental imperatives is the optimal method for treating suicidal adolescents and their families in a brief treatment context.

Two Central Principles

Given the limited scope of this chapter, however, it is not possible to describe the rationales and treatment approaches used in the ADSP in full. Therefore, we will focus upon two central principles frequently employed in treatment in the clinic. Simply put, these are: (1) the rate of development (that is, the speed at which separation and individuation occur), and whether the adolescent and the family are in synchrony regarding the rate of this process, are often components of a problem which requires resolution (see also Boscolo, Cecchin, Hoffman, & Penn, 1987; Gustafson, 1986); and (2) a suicide attempt in adolescence can be understood as a problem-solving behavior (see also Orbach, 1986, 1988). In particular, the impact of the first principle is to cause the adolescent to feel that the problem which demands resolution in fact *has no solution;* this dilemma leads to suicide as an attempt to solve such an "insolvable problem." Thus, these two principles are closely allied, and will be addressed concurrently.

The "Rate-of-Development" Principle

We often use the following metaphor, or a variant of it, in helping adolescents and their families to understand the synchrony or asynchrony of the speed of separation and individuation (the "rate-of-development" principle):

> Imagine the family of an adolescent as a group of people who have chosen to take a long trip together in separate cars, such that each individual is in control of his or her own vehicle. In taking the trip, they have intended to travel as a "caravan"; that is, to keep pace with each other such that no one moves too far ahead or too fast, and no one lags behind or gives up altogether. However, in the midst of the trip, there are various times when one or more members of the group speed up, threatening to leave others in the dust. This gives the others the choice either to speed up as well, to slow down, or to maintain speed in the hope that the speeders will recognize this and slow down; their other choice is to leave the caravan, pull off the highway, and travel on alone. Alternatively, some members may suddenly slow down, requiring others to decelerate as well, or to risk moving too far ahead if they maintain speed. Further, there are times when a member of the group may turn off the road for some reason, requiring the others to search for him or her. Finally, there is the unfortunate possibility that the vehicle of one of the members of the caravan may break down or crash, leading to the need for emergency measures.

This highway metaphor illustrates effectively the ways in which adolescents and their families can be seen as a system in development, with each individual needing to evolve in synchrony with the others for equilibrium to be maintained. Clearly, one or another family member sometimes moves at a faster rate than the others, causing a crisis to occur. There are several ways in which this can be manifested: First of all, the adolescent may be moving too quickly into adult choices and peer activities for the parents, or the adolescent may feel that the parents are expecting him or her to take on adult responsibilities prematurely. Second, an adolescent may feel the need to slow progress, refusing to participate in normal, expected activities such as school and social interactions. Third, he or she may feel so constrained by family pressures that opting out of the developmental process entirely seems like the only plausible choice.

In addition, successful negotiation of the developmental tasks of adolescence can be impeded by open wounds or damage, such as the sequelae of physical or sexual abuse, adversarial relationships between parents, and so on. Finally, adolescents sometimes are not sure that their parents are ready for their departure or that the marriage will survive; likewise, parents are not always secure in the feeling that their children are equipped to move into relationships beyond the family.

These scenarios all relate to the "rate-of-development" principle. It is quite apparent that there are a number of ways in which an adolescent and his or her parents could feel at odds with each other, and that problems could arise easily. Often these problems can pit the adolescent's forward movement into adulthood against his or her desires to remain a child and be nurtured. In addition, there can be circumstances in which the adolescent feels pulled in two directions at once by conflicting messages from parents, either between the parents or within each of them.

"Insolvable" Problems

Such circumstances can engender the feeling in adolescents that their current problems are insurmountable. What we would like to suggest is that a suicide attempt in adolescence frequently can be understood as an attempt to solve a problem with developmental overtones that is experienced as having no solution. We have observed time and again that adolescents who make suicide attempts experience themselves as being in circumstances from which there is no clear path to extrication, and that the suicide attempt is at least in part a way of resolving this dilemma. In general, these "insolvable problems" (Orbach, 1986, 1988) appear related to the rate-of-development principle.

Case Example

Seventeen-year-old Roseanne, the youngest of four children in an intact Irish/Italian family, was referred to the ADSP after her second suicide attempt in as many years. Her parents had a long history of marital discord, and Roseanne and her mother were highly enmeshed. When Roseanne made strides toward a life independent of her mother, her mother objected. For her part, Roseanne worried a great deal about her mother, who had a history of suicidal behavior as well; she was unsure whether her parents' marriage would survive when she left home, or whether her mother would survive at all. Loyal to her mother, Roseanne stayed home a great deal, but became increasingly depressed; she felt torn between her desire to move on with her life and her mother's implicit demand that she remain her "baby." Faced with this "insolvable problem," she ingested a number of pills and went to sleep, informing no one of her action until the following day.

In circumstances such as those facing Roseanne, the suicidal adolescent experiences developmental dilemmas as unresolvable: In essence, he or she feels that it is not possible to grow up without significant loss or betrayal, nor is it possible to stay a child without significant loss or betrayal. Growing up implies the loss of protection and nurturance that the family can provide; staying a child implies the loss of the prerogatives of adulthood and the potential to discover and explore one's capabilities.

Separation Within Connectedness

Although apparently insolvable, these developmental dilemmas are in fact not without resolution, but they do call for flexibility. This requires the understanding that compromises must be made, that losses will inevitably be incurred while gains are solidified. In order to evolve into a fully functioning adult, an adolescent does need to move away from the family, which implies a loss of the kind of connectedness that prevails in earlier life (Garcia Preto, 1988; Garcia Preto & Travis, 1985). However, as is suggested by more recent writings on adolescent development (Apter, 1990; Fishman, 1988), healthy evolution in the family does not require that adolescents and their parents disengage entirely. In fact, for both the adolescent and the family, separation and individuation can occur and flourish within a context of connectedness. In this way, the adolescent and his or her parents are able to create a more flexible relationship that will allow for further personal and systemic growth without rupture and isolated disengagement.

Case Example

Elsie, who was the youngest of three children in a traditional Puerto Rican family, was significantly depressed. After her second suicide attempt, she expressed concerns about her parents' fragile marriage and her anticipation of "growing up and being alone." As a result, her parents moved Elsie's bed into their bedroom, where her mother could keep a closer watch on her. This sleeping arrangement, which appeared protective of Elsie, also precluded any intimacy between her parents. In couples' sessions, Elsie's parents were helped to communicate more effectively, working through some of their resentments and disappointments. Consequently, they became willing to move Elsie back to her own room. When this was presented to her, however, Elsie "put on the brakes," feeling left out and rejected. In subsequent individual and family sessions, treatment focused on developing a more flexible, age-appropriate relationship between Elsie and her mother, so that they could function separately while maintaining the positive connectedness of their mother-daughter relationship.

The task of separating while maintaining connectedness is difficult to attain, however. When the adolescent has needed to slam on the brakes in order to alter a rate of development that was intolerable, the pace of development in the family often moves into retrograde. Adolescent and parents alike feel manipulated, controlled, or intruded upon, their needs and feelings disregarded (Zimmerman, 1991; Zimmerman & Zayas, in press). Movement through time has stopped for such a family (Garcia Preto, 1988).

Consequently, in order to access the developmental derailment in the family system as a whole and to remove the onus from one or another family member, therapeutic intervention often is required. One way we frequently address this need is to reframe the struggle between parents and adolescent in terms of the speed at which development is occurring and what various members of the system are doing in order to regulate it.

Case Example

In the Vasquez family, the parents espoused relatively traditional Latino values. They felt that their three adolescent daughters were moving too fast, getting involved in peer activities and sexual behavior for which they were too young. The girls felt that their parents were not able to understand them, could not see that their behavior was not meant as disrespectful or rebellious, but was more an expression of the experimentation that adolescents normatively go through. The daughters' way of expressing this concretely was to refuse to get out of bed in the morning; all three missed numerous days of school this way. Following a couples' session, the parents began to attend more to their relationship separate from their children, apparently taking to heart the idea that their daughters would move on into adulthood and that they needed to focus on how their lives would be after their children were gone. In turn, the daughters were able to articulate their feelings and were able to get on with their lives in school.

However, as things seemed to be improving, the middle daughter, Iris, reported this incident: One night after 11 P.M., she repeatedly entered her parents' bedroom in order to retrieve one or another thing she claimed she needed (such as a hairbrush); her parents finally "kicked [her] out." As a result, she felt she was being thrown out of the nest; in a family session, she said, "They're going to leave me, they don't care anymore." In response, the therapist suggested that her parents' choice to move on with their lives might have made her feel that they were going too fast for her, that she wasn't ready for this change yet. This intervention, and others like it, allows all members of the family to become aware of the concept of the speed of development. As a result, they can make more conscious and informed choices about the rate at which they can agree to move ahead.

TECHNICAL ISSUES

The treatment approach we employ, although often effective, requires that certain technical issues be considered carefully. These include: (1) approaches to transference manifestations; (2) issues regarding confidentiality; (3) direct exposure of adolescents to toxic parental attitudes; and (4) potential dilution of family work through addressing family issues in separate individual sessions.

Transference Manifestations

Several authors have expressed the concern that, in using a single therapist for individual and family treatment, the transference may be less fully developed or less intense than it would be in individual treatment alone (Charny, 1966; Glick, Clarkin, & Kessler, 1987). Although this may be the case if one were intent upon allowing a classical transference to develop, our treatment is offered over a short period of time. In such brief treatment contexts, a number of authors have suggested that transference manifestations should be interpreted or confronted as soon as they arise so that they will not become central to treatment (Alexander & French, 1946; Mann, 1973; Sifneos, 1979). Therefore, we position ourselves as the "family's" therapist so that we may allow the family (as a group and as individuals) to develop a more systemic transference to us as facilitators of their growth.

Confidentiality

Managing confidentiality in the context of treatment that integrates individual and family modalities is not a simple task. In general, our approach is to delineate in the initial appointment with the family the limits to confidentiality regarding risk to self or others, or current physical or sexual abuse. In addition, we make it clear that treatment-destructive secrets cannot be kept by the therapist. However, there are instances in which information is told to us in a session with a subunit of the family that we do not feel is necessary to bring to light in a family session.

Case Example

Anna, age 15, reported in an individual session that she had been sexually abused as an eight-year-old by a maternal aunt. She stated that she was not ready to discuss this experience with her family, feeling concerned about the consequences. Since the abuse was not current, the choice was made to respect her wishes. Simultaneously, the therapist offered Anna help in disclosing this to the family if she chose to do so in the future.

In another case, however, the choice was made to inform the family of a confidential issue.

Case Example

Debbie, age 18, had a history of drug and alcohol abuse along with several serious suicide attempts. In an individual session, she revealed that she had begun drinking again and had lied to her parents about it. The therapist explained that this information could not be kept confidential because of the potential risk to Debbie. Although she initially resisted, Debbie was willing to share this with her parents with the help of the therapist. Her parents responded in a supportive way, and her father, a recovered alcoholic himself, was identified as an "expert" in this area. His help was solicited in monitoring Debbie's behavior. This intervention improved the relationship between father and daughter, and also brought the father into the family system in a more active way. His self-esteem and sense of efficacy grew as a result.

Toxic Attitudes

Some authors have expressed concern about the "traumatic effects on children of being explicitly confronted with implicit dangers in their intrafamilial relationships—such as the hostile, rejecting feelings of a parent" (Malone, 1979, p. 4). However, it is our experience that it is often better to bring these issues to light so that they can be managed therapeutically, especially in the aftermath of a suicide attempt. In fact, frequently the adolescent has already intuited the parent's feelings, and these feelings actually become less destructive when they can be expressed in a controlled environment such as the therapist's office.

Case Example

In the Vasquez family, described earlier, the oldest daughter, Anna, had become pregnant out of wedlock and suffered a miscarriage early in treatment. Although Anna's pregnancy was deeply disturbing to her parents, they did not express their feelings directly; rather, the issue was partially revealed in cryptic side comments. In family sessions, the therapist encouraged the parents to express their disappointment more openly, which they proceeded to do. This culminated in a dramatic session in which Anna screamed at her parents that they could not possibly understand her and that she desperately missed her baby. She was then comforted by her younger sister and, more tentatively, by her mother. In subsequent sessions, all family members were able to articulate their ambivalent feelings about her pregnancy and other behavior, and a stronger, more positive bond was reformed between Anna and her parents.

Dilution of Intensity

Finally, some authors suggest that the intensity of family issues may be diluted if they are raised in individual sessions (e.g., Fishman, 1988). However, we have found that it is often in such individual sessions that issues can be more fully expressed initially. In fact, this is sometimes the only context in which an adolescent will reveal certain thoughts and feelings at all. Likewise, in separate sessions, parents may feel freer to speak more objectively about their roles as parents (Garcia Preto, 1988). Again, as is the case with unspoken toxic feelings, therapeutic leverage can be gained by exploring such concerns in the controlled context of the treatment room. As a result of such exploration, these concerns can be clarified with the adolescent or the parents without the confusion, distraction, and emotional intensity that sometimes ensue in family sessions. Subsequently, once the issues have been articulated in individual or subsystem meetings, they can be brought to the family with the assistance of the therapist, to the greater benefit of all concerned.

Case Example

Roseanne, mentioned earlier, remained sullen and withdrawn in family sessions, unwilling to reveal the reasons for her suicide attempts. In an individual session, however, she admitted feeling that she was a burden to her family and that they would be better off without her. With encouragement, she chose to allow the therapist to use this information in a family session, although she was unable to do so herself. When informed, her parents were surprised and upset, but responded empathically; her mother, generally stoic and resistant, cried when she imagined her life without Roseanne. In addition to opening up new and positive lines of family communication, the revelation of Roseanne's feelings allowed her siblings to share similar ones.

CONCLUSION

In conclusion, we have presented some theoretical perspectives and technical issues regarding an integrative approach to the treatment of suicidal adolescents and their families in a brief treatment context. We have suggested that the dynamics of the "insolvable problem" and the rate of development of the adolescent and family are often central in such cases. Consequently, our approach to treatment integrates family systems, developmental, and psychodynamic theoretical perspectives in a technical combination of individual and family modalities, which can be effective in treating suicidal adolescents. Ultimately, such an approach can allow the family as a system to move ahead at a mutually acceptable rate of speed. What can be achieved is a successful renegotiation of relationships that allows the adolescent to move into adulthood while retaining connectedness with the family. This renegotiation also allows the family to experience individuation within the context of strong interpersonal bonds.

REFERENCES

Alexander, F., & French, T. M. (1946). *Psychoanalytic therapy: Principles and applications.* New York: Ronald Press.

Apter, T. (1990). *Altered loves.* New York: St. Martin's Press.

Arkowitz, H. (1991). Introductory statement: Psychotherapy integration comes of age. *Journal of Psychotherapy Integration, 1*(1), 1–3.

Beitman, B. D., Goldfried, M. R., & Norcross, J. C. (1989). The movement toward integrating the psychotherapies: An overview. *American Journal of Psychiatry, 146*(2), 138–147.

Boscolo, L., Cecchin, G., Hoffman, L., & Penn, P. (1987). *Milan systemic family therapy: Conversations in theory and practice.* New York: Basic Books.

Carter, C. (1987). Some indications for combining individual and family therapy. *American Journal of Family Therapy, 15*(2), 99–110.

Case, E. M., & Robinson, N. S. (1990). Toward integration: The changing world of family therapy. *American Journal of Family Therapy, 18*(2), 153–160.

Charny, I. W. (1966). Integrated individual and family psychotherapy. *Family Process, 5*(2), 179–198.

Feldman, L. B. (1985). Integrative multi-level therapy: A comprehensive interpersonal and intrapsychic approach. *Journal of Marriage and Family Therapy, 11,* 357–372.

Feldman, L. B., & Powell, S. L. (1992). Integrating therapeutic modalities. In J. C. Norcross & M. R. Goldfried (Eds.), *Handbook of Psychotherapy Integration* (pp. 503–532). New York: Basic Books.

Fishman, H. C. (1988). *Treating troubled adolescents: A family therapy approach.* New York: Basic Books.

Garcia Preto, N. (1988). Transformation of the family system in adolescence. In B. Carter & M. McGoldrick (Eds.), *The changing family life cycle: A framework for family therapy* (2nd ed.) (pp. 255–283). New York: Gardner Press.

Garcia Preto, N., & Travis, N. (1985). The adolescent phase of the family life cycle. In M. P. Mirkin & S. L. Koman (Eds.), *Handbook of adolescents and family therapy* (pp. 21–38). New York: Gardner Press.

Glick, I., Clarkin, J., & Kessler, D. (1987). *Marital and family therapy* (3rd ed.). Orlando, FL: Gruner Stratton.

Guerney, L., & Guerney, B. (1987). Integrating child and family therapy. *Psychotherapy, 24*(3S), 609–614.

Gustafson, J. P. (1986). *The complex secret of brief psychotherapy*. New York: Norton.

Haley, J. (1987). The disappearance of the individual. *Family Therapy Networker, 11*, 39–40.

Kaffman, M. (1965). Family diagnosis and therapy in child emotional pathology. *Family Process, 4*, 241–258.

Karasu, T. B. (1979). Toward unification of psychotherapies: A complementary model. *American Journal of Psychotherapy, 33*(4), 555–563.

Kaslow, N. J., & Racusin, G. R. (1990). Family therapy or child therapy: An open or shut case. *Journal of Family Psychology, 3*(3), 273–289.

Kirschner, D. A., & Kirschner, S. (1986). *Comprehensive family therapy: An integration of systemic and psychodynamic treatment models*. New York: Brunner/Mazel.

Kirschner, S., & Kirschner, D. A. (1990). Comprehensive family therapy: Integrating individual, marital, and family therapy. In F. Kaslow (Ed.), *Voices in family psychology* (vol. 2, pp. 231–243). San Francisco, CA: Sage.

Landau-Stanton, J., & Stanton, M. D. (1985). Treating suicidal adolescents and their families. In M. P. Mirkin & S. L. Koman (Eds.), *Handbook of adolescents and family therapy* (pp. 309–328). New York: Gardner Press.

Lazarus, A., & Messer, S. (1991). Does chaos prevail? An exchange on technical eclecticism and assimilative integration. *Journal of Psychotherapy Integration, 1*(2), 143–158.

Levant, R. F., & Haffey, N. A. (1981). Toward an integration of child and family therapy. *International Journal of Family Therapy, Summer*, 130–142.

Malone, C. A. (1979). Child psychiatry and family therapy: An overview. *Journal of the American Academy of Child Psychiatry, 18*, 4–20.

Mann, J. (1973). *Time-limited psychotherapy*. Cambridge, MA: Harvard University Press.

Nichols, M. (1987). The individual in the system. *Family Therapy Networker, 11*, 33–38.

Norcross, J. C., & Grencavage, L. M. (1989). Eclecticism and integration in counseling and psychotherapy: Major themes and obstacles. *British Journal of Guidance Counseling, 17*, 227–247.

Orbach, I. (1986). The "insolvable problem" as a determinant in the dynamics of suicidal behavior in children. *Journal of American Psychotherapy, 40*(4), 511–520.

Orbach, I. (1988). *Children who don't want to live.* San Francisco, CA: Jossey-Bass.

Pinsof, W. M. (1983). Integrative problem-centered therapy: Toward the synthesis of family and individual psychotherapies. *Journal of Marriage and Family Therapy, 9,* 19–35.

Pfeffer, C. R. (1989). Life stress and family risk factors for youth fatal and nonfatal suicidal behavior. In C. R. Pfeffer, (Ed.), *Suicide among youth: Perspectives on risk and prevention* (pp. 143–164). Washington, DC: American Psychiatric Press.

Shaffer, D. (1974). Suicide in childhood and early adolescence. *Journal of Child Psychology and Psychiatry, 15,* 275–291.

Shafii, M., Carrigan, S., Whittinghill, J. R., & Derrick, A. (1985). Psychological autopsy of completed suicide in children and adolescents. *American Journal of Psychiatry, 142,* 1061–1064.

Sifneos, P. E. (1979). *Short-term dynamic psychotherapy.* New York: Plenum.

Spirito, A., Brown, L., Overholser, J., & Fritz, G. (1989). Attempted suicide in adolescence: A review and critique of the literature. *Clinical Psychology Review, 9,* 335–363.

Tishler, C. L., McKenry, P. C., & Morgan, K. C. (1981). Adolescent suicide attempts: Some significant factors. *Suicide and Life-Threatening Behavior, 11,* 86–92.

Turgay, A. (1989). An integrative treatment approach to child and adolescent suicidal behavior. *Psychiatric Clinics of North America, 12*(4), 971–985.

Vane, J. R., & DeMaria, T. (1988). The psychologist as general family practitioner. *Professional Psychology: Research and Practice, 19*(1), 118–120.

Wachtel, P. L. (1991). From eclecticism to synthesis: Toward a more seamless psychotherapeutic integration. *Journal of Psychotherapy Integration, 1*(1), 43–54.

Wachtel, P. L., & Wachtel, E. F. (1986). *Family dynamics in individual psychotherapy: A guide to clinical strategies.* New York: Guilford Press.

Zimmerman, J. K. (1991). Crossing the desert alone: An etiological model of female adolescent suicidality. In C. Gilligan, A. G. Rogers, & D. L. Tolman, (Eds.), *Women, girls, and psychotherapy: Reframing resistance* (pp. 223–241). New York: Haworth Press.

Zimmerman, J. K., & Zayas, L. H. (in press). Suicidal adolescent Latinas: Culture, female development, and restoring the mother-daughter relationship. In S. S. Canetto & D. Lester (Eds.), *Women and suicide: A feminist perspective.* New York: Springer.

10

Group Treatment of Suicidal Adolescents

SETH ARONSON AND
SAUL SCHEIDLINGER

This chapter deals with the uniquely challenging problem of utilizing the group modality to treat suicidal adolescents. The importance of group life in personality development has been detailed elsewhere (Grunebaum & Solomon, 1982). The normative peer group takes on a pivotal role in adolescence where it becomes a necessary stepping-stone away from the family. It also serves as the laboratory for testing one's identity, intimacy, social skills, and budding sexuality. As noted by Blos (1967), the group bond allows for a "second individuation" consistent with the adolescent's need to distinguish between the idealized parents of childhood and the real parents of today. The group's support in the face of teenagers' ever-present self-doubt, shame, guilt, and loneliness is proverbial.

We have noted in a previous publication how these motivational factors for change and growth have been widely utilized in the group treatment of disturbed adolescents (Scheidlinger & Aronson, 1991). In fact, with a few exceptions, group therapy has come to be widely viewed as the treatment of choice for most psychologically impaired adolescents (Scheidlinger, 1985). How then can one explain the unusually sparse literature and practice in employing the group modality for suicidal adolescents in clinical contexts? The likely major reasons are: fear of "contagion," which is an ever-present concern in schools where suicides have occurred; a view that suicide is a "private" matter, not readily shared in a group; and insufficient numbers of trained group therapists. This will be further discussed in the "Special Problems" section later.

189

CHARACTERISTICS OF
SUICIDAL ADOLESCENTS

Adolescent suicide has become a highly publicized issue in recent years. Given the marked increase in suicides among 15- to 24-year-olds, many researchers have investigated the risk factors as well as prevention and treatment programs (Shaffer, Garland, Gould, Fisher, & Trautman, 1988).

The results of many of these studies, most notably those of Shaffer and associates (1988) and Brent (Brent et al., 1986; Brent et al., 1988), indicate that adolescent suicidal behavior is not a unitary phenomenon but is rather associated with several risk factors and with various types of psychopathology. These risk factors include some degree of substance use, a history of impulsive and/or aggressive behavior, and the suicide or attempted suicide of a family member, among others.

In addition, Pfeffer's (1986) description of suicidal youth has included such characteristics as:

- *Poor peer relationships* due to inadequate socialization skills. At a point when they need to bond with contemporaries, these youngsters often are rebuffed by peers and lack the wherewithal to attempt to make connections outside the home. They continue searching for new figures with whom to identify but are unable to make contact. These difficulties with peers often contribute to low self-esteem, as a negative self-image is reinforced continually.

- *Cognitive distortions,* including the irrational belief that they are defective, inadequate, or unworthy. These distortions include a tendency to interpret events in a persistently negative way.

- *Deficient coping patterns.* These patients also have little awareness of their feeling state, especially of growing angry. Their frustration tolerance is quite low, as is their threshold for anxiety. When they become angry or anxious, it is intensely experienced and they feel that they have no recourse other than self-injurious behaviors.

- *Pathological ego defenses.* Pathological introjection, repression, denial, projection, and somatization are utilized by these patients in an effort to ward off painful affects. Poor boundary differentiation between the patient and his or her family has been noted as well. As a result, there are often intense symbiotic relationships within the family.

- *Family dysfunction.* As noted, there are often symbiotic enmeshments within the family as well as chaotic turmoil, as the adolescent attempts unsuccessfully to disengage from the family. Anecdotal accounts of precipitating events prior to suicide attempts often point to a conflict with the parents, a dispute with the family over a boyfriend or girlfriend, and school failure.

Group therapy offers an opportunity to address each of these issues in a milieu that is developmentally syntonic and perhaps more acceptable to the adolescent than individual or family treatment. However, it calls for special care that the group constitutes a safe and trustworthy environment from the very beginning.

PLANNING AND MANAGEMENT OF GROUPS

Because there are logistical differences in planning for groups on an inpatient service, we will focus here on groups for suicidal adolescents conducted in an outpatient setting only.

In planning for therapy groups for suicidal adolescents, there are many issues to consider. These include, among others, physical setting and context, therapist characteristics, comprehensive referral system, and inclusion criteria.

Physical Setting and Context

The physical setting and context are important. Thus, Motto (1990) advocated that such groups be run under the auspices of some organizational sponsor, such as a hospital, clinic, or social service agency. This provides for the needed backup and support. Arrangements for such support are critical as the suicidal adolescents should feel that they have access to a therapist at all times. The backup may take the form of a 24-hour answering service or simply the availability of a psychiatric emergency room.

Therapist Characteristics

It takes a special blend of therapist characteristics to treat such a difficult and anxiety-evoking population. Therapists working with suicidal adolescents should have confronted personal anxieties and concerns regarding death and suicide lest their own issues inhibit discussion or make the group setting one in which several topics seem "forbidden." A therapist working with adolescents must be especially honest, direct and genuine, and able to guide the group toward an atmosphere of safety and trust. Furthermore, empathy and care must be communicated. An active stance on the part of the therapist is also crucial in working with adolescents; they do not appreciate nor will they stand for undue permissiveness or for a silent stance on the part of the adult. This is especially true of younger adolescent boys who are best reached via activities and games. The group therapist must be willing to withstand and contain the provocativeness and "testing" for which adolescents are so well known; at the same time, there is need for the direct and firm setting of appropriate limits. Last, it is important that the therapist be trained in the theory of group therapy and have a solid working knowledge of child and adolescent development. Ongoing supervision is a "must."

At our clinic at the Bronx Municipal Hospital Center, we use a cotherapy model with a male and female cotherapist, as advocated by Davis and Lohr (1971). A cotherapy model provides support to the therapists, helps to minimize problems in emergency situations, and allows for continuity if one of the therapists is absent. The use of male and female cotherapists also enhances the idea of the group being a "corrective emotional experience" as a more positive family environment.

Comprehensive Referral System

In the best possible circumstances, a comprehensive system for referral to the group needs to be in place. Once patients are referred, they should be screened by the cotherapists. The purpose of the screening is to establish at least a minimal working alliance with the patient, as well as to prepare him or her for the initial questions and concerns regarding joining a group (Scheidlinger, 1985). It is generally at the screening that questions arise regarding confidentiality, who the other members will be, family involvement, and the purpose of the group. The screening also should be used to assess the severity of suicidal risk of the potential group member. Obviously, those adolescents who are acutely suicidal and at imminent risk may require a more structured environment.

Inclusion Criteria

Each patient should be carefully considered for inclusion in the group. Slavson (1950) has written of "balancing" groups—that is, providing for an equilibrium of ethnic, racial, psychosocial, and educational characteristics. Levels of sophistication and life experience are important as well. Care should be given toward balancing the number of boys and girls in the group also. Ideally, one should aim for eight to ten members.

In working with middle to older adolescents, a coed group best affords the opportunity for learning social skills and experiencing interaction with members of the opposite sex.

In general, teens tend to be more amenable to joining a group to discuss general problems, or what to do when one feels depressed, rather than a group explicitly labeled "For Those at Risk for Suicide." Because it is such an emotionally charged concept, the idea of suicide will remain in the background and come to the fore when an acceptable degree of trust and safety is experienced in the group.

In fact, research suggests that *suicide prevention groups* per se—addressed to general student populations—are in some cases counterproductive (Garland, Shaffer, & Whittle, 1989; Shaffer, Garland, Vieland, Underwood, & Busner, 1991). In contrast, Scheidlinger (1985) has found "rap" groups, focusing on psychosocial stressors to which adolescents are prone, where the subject of suicide is discussed in tandem with other problems (such as peer relationships or family difficulties) to be more successful. At our clinic, presenting the group as a "rap group" or a chance to talk with other adolescents about common problems and issues has worked well.

The question of time-limited versus open-ended groups is one that has become particularly salient today, with the advent of managed care. The San Mateo program (Ross & Motto, 1984), as well as the one at Langley-Porter (Asimos & Rosen, 1978), which worked with suicidal adults, began with a time limit but found it necessary to extend the duration of the group due to clinical considerations. We have found a trial time-limited period of 12 weeks, with an option to reevaluate continuation of the group at that juncture, to be helpful. In this way, the adolescents do not feel they are committing themselves to some indefinite treatment; however, at the same time, if they find it valuable, the option to continue is available. A trial period also tends to bind the adolescent's anxiety about dependency and independence.

THERAPEUTIC FACTORS IN THE GROUP THERAPY OF SUICIDAL ADOLESCENTS

Yalom (1975) has outlined therapeutic factors necessary for group work, such as universality, instillation of hope, cohesion, interpersonal learning, and recapitulation of the primary family group. Many of these are particularly relevant in addressing the issues of suicidal adolescents.

A major curative factor mentioned by Yalom is universality. The notion that everyone in the group is "in the same boat" provides comfort and support and decreases the sense of isolation a depressed, suicidal adolescent may feel.

At the first meeting of one of our groups the adolescent girls were quiet and shy, eyes cast downward. They quickly offered names and schools they attended as a means of introduction and then were silent. Suddenly, Annie, a gregarious Jamaican girl, blurted out, "I was thrown out of my house this weekend by my stepfather." Blanca replied, "You have fights with your stepfather too?" This commonality quickly set the group at ease.

Adolescence is filled with self-consciousness, and being in a group with peers who have similar difficulties is reassuring. This helps to decrease the sense of loneliness and isolation. Feeling comfortable among empathic peers, the adolescent group member then may feel safer to explore more openly those issues that were previously too painful to address. We have found it successful to use poetry and music as a way to engage the adolescents, while helping to stimulate discussion of troubling feelings and issues. We have shown such movies as *Purple Rain* and *The Breakfast Club,* which deal with family conflict, physical abuse, and suicidality. This has led to some very candid discussions of these issues. In addition, we encourage the group members to bring in tapes or poems that they feel are relevant and want to share with the other members. We found that this helps suicidal adolescents address more complex issues in a nonthreatening way, while concurrently fostering a sense of responsibility for the group (and ultimately, themselves).

In the give-and-take of group sessions, stressors and precipitants to suicidal feelings can be identified. Many suicidal adolescents have underdeveloped "signal anxiety"—that is, they are unable to modulate effectively their affective responses to stress. Their peers can help by highlighting stressors of their own; commonalities in their experience are then readily discovered. Once these stressors have been identified, the group can begin to establish a hierarchy of coping strategies ranging from (at the least effective and productive end of the continuum) self-injurious behavior, substance abuse, and running away, through arguing with a person who has upset them, to (at the productive end of the continuum) getting help from support systems such as the group leaders or fellow members. The therapist should help to foster verbal expression of the adolescent's feelings while suppressing any physical expression. Reflection before acting on feelings is encouraged in an effort to develop the adolescent's self-awareness about and sensitivity to stressful issues.

Case Example

Maritza had been briefly hospitalized for ingesting pills following an argument with her mother. The group helped her to develop alternative coping strategies for dealing with her anxiety after these arguments, such as leaving the house, calling a friend, or listening to her favorite calming music.

The group also provides an arena in which the impact of one's behavior on others can be explored. Perceptions of self and others for these patients are often fraught with conflict and doubt. Once comfortable in the group, the members may give feedback to others about their behavior and receive feedback as well. Some group therapists have used role-playing techniques to enhance such interactions. Feedback can help modify an adolescent's more aggressive, impulsive response to frustration or disappointment. In listening to others in the group, adolescents may compare their reactions to a peer's situation and perhaps see other options for themselves in problematic circumstances and dilemmas.

Case Example

In one session, Samantha was discussing how angry she gets at her boyfriend. After a previous argument, she had taken an overdose of pills. Samantha said she was angry and hurt by her boyfriend's recent actions. Luann asked if Samantha had told him how hurt she was. Samantha said she hadn't. Luann said, "I think you should tell him—he's the reason for your being mad. Don't keep it in." Later, Luann commented on how she often keeps her anger to herself and perhaps it would be better if *she* told people how angry she was.

Ideally, the group members should begin to give up some of their defensive use of externalization and blaming. Gradually the adolescents begin to assume more responsibility for their actions which, in turn, also serves to enhance self-esteem. Supportive feedback from group members also helps to nurture a healthier sense of self with a resultant increase in positive self-regard. This is a major treatment goal for depressed, suicidal youth.

The male-female cotherapy team provides healthy role models with whom the group members can identify. Many suicidal adolescents came from dysfunctional families in which pathological identifications are formed. The therapists represent new adults whom the adolescents may observe. Ideally, as a result of the observation process, the adolescents will begin to incorporate some of the more positive aspects of the therapists (and group).

Case Example

Janine noted how calm one of the therapists seemed. She asked him, "Don't you ever get so mad that you punch a wall? I always do." The therapist explained that, like all people, he got angry, but used words to express his feelings. Janine began to wonder aloud if she couldn't learn to be less physically explosive when upset.

In addition, Scheidlinger (1974) has discussed the concept of the "mother group"; the group-as-a-whole may be viewed unconsciously as a positive, need-gratifying maternal image.

The Langley-Porter program (Billings, Rosen, Asimos, & Motto, 1974) stressed the need for group members to deal consciously and effectively with their anger. The therapists felt that in order for the members not to "act out" their anger, they need to develop a conscious awareness of what makes them angry (as seen in the preceding vignette of Samantha and Luann). Once this is achieved, the patients then can learn about the defensive operations that block the expression of this rage. Finally, the members may use the group as an in vivo experience, testing out angry responses while learning that there is no threat to self-esteem and group membership if anger is displayed. Comments by the therapists such as "you may get angry here and we might not agree, but it doesn't mean you are not valued and liked as a group member" help support these therapeutic gains.

Many theorists have described the various developmental stages of adolescent groups (Garland, Jones, & Kolodny, 1973). For a time-limited focused group, the work can be divided roughly into a beginning, middle, and end phase. Initially, the adolescents may be shy and hesitant with each other and mistrustful of the adult leaders. Once trust is established, common themes such as difficulties in family and peer relationships, loss and grief, pathological response to pain and frustration (such as suicidal gestures and feelings), and how to cope with these problems are addressed. In the final phase, termination is discussed. Termination can be a particularly sensitive issue for suicidal adolescents as many of them have responded to perceived rejection and abandonment with a suicide attempt; nevertheless, during adolescence, they must necessarily go through a process of separation and termination. Helping these troubled adolescents master a successful termination without responding impulsively can be most beneficial at times.

Case Example

Troy, an outgoing 17-year-old boy, had great difficulty addressing the termination of the group. In the weeks preceding the final session, he often changed the subject when the topic of termination arose. In the final session, he was able to acknowledge his difficulty and disclosed that in all his previous therapies, he had left precipitously, avoiding saying good-bye. The group, he felt, had provided him with enough support and friends that he felt he could stay in touch with members and the therapists. This made ending more tolerable for him.

INDICATIONS AND CONTRAINDICATIONS

During the screening interviews, the therapists should consider the balancing of the group as well as the group's composition. Those patients who are psychotic or violence-prone should not be included. Many suicidal adolescents have substance abuse problems. Their difficulty with drugs and alcohol may be a central issue requiring their involvement in a drug treatment program, or it may represent an attempt to flee a stressful life situation. Careful screening by the therapists can help decide proper placement.

Many outpatient groups for suicidal adolescents require the adolescent to be in individual treatment as well. This provides more support (for both therapist and patient) as well as serving as a complement to input from the group session. Individual sessions often allow a slower process of working through and mastering the therapeutic gains of the group. In our experience, we have found that individual treatment is an important adjunct to group work. Each group member, if not already in individual therapy, is assigned an individual therapist (Scheidlinger & Porter, 1980).

Group treatment also may provide support for a suicidal adolescent who is in conjoint family therapy and who is reluctant or unable to confront painful issues within the family. Often, through role-playing and support in the group, adolescents gain the courage to express thoughts and feelings during family sessions that they were previously unable to do so.

SPECIAL PROBLEMS

Working with suicidal adolescents requires the careful negotiation of a myriad of issues. The anxiety around grouping suicidal patients into one unit has been well documented in the literature. Farberow and Schneidman (1961) have discussed the commonly held myth that if one talks with suicidal patients about suicide, it will cause them actually to kill themselves. Hackel and Asimos (1981) have described the enormous logistical difficulties they encountered in beginning groups for suicidal patients. Often the sponsoring agency balks or resists because of fear of contagion of suicidal behavior. In setting up such a group, then, care should be taken calmly to allay administrators' fears regarding this treatment modality. The combination of individual and group therapy discussed earlier (Scheidlinger & Porter, 1980) often helps an administrative staff to feel reassured that there is a "safety net."

The therapists who run such groups must be well trained in developmental issues of adolescence, crisis intervention, and group therapy techniques. Leading a group for suicidal adolescents can be a daunting task, with tremendous demands put on the cotherapists. These cotherapists must be prepared to deal with (at times) extremely needy teenagers, who simultaneously may pull out an arsenal of insults and provocations designed to keep the therapists at bay. The therapists must be careful not to take these insults and provocations personally and also must not step into an omnipotent role, encouraging too much dependency on the part of the suicidal adolescent. The group therapists must realize that they cannot rescue all the patients and that, eventually, the adolescents must assume some responsibility for living. It is important that group therapists be tolerant, noncritical, open, and comfortable with themselves. Often adolescent patients ask personal questions that feel invasive and unsettling; group therapists need to handle this with relative ease. Care must be taken not to overidentify with the adolescent's plight; on the other hand, adolescents generally will experience an overemphasis on conformity as being too much like a parent. The other danger in working with needy adolescents resides in being too seductive with them. Suicidal adolescents are at a most vulnerable point and can easily be led to gratify some need of group therapists. Overprotecting suicidal patients as a "conscious" result of wanting to care for them may serve to collude with their feelings of helplessness and should be carefully monitored.

A problem particular to this kind of group is the case of a suicide or suicide attempt by a group member. Should this occur, it is imperative to address it in an honest, forthright fashion. The therapists must be genuine in the expression of their feelings; otherwise, the group members may feel that the therapists' silence is an endorsement of emotional distancing, numbing, and isolation. Often group members (and therapists) feel guilt and personal failure at not having "recognized the warning signs" and "saved" the member. They may have an increase in suicidal feelings, but it is important to deal directly with the issues of loss and anger while providing support to the other members. While a suicide is a most tragic occurrence, such an event can lead to a keener awareness of what it means to be left behind as a survivor.

SUMMARY AND RECOMMENDATIONS FOR FUTURE WORK

Group therapy for suicidal adolescents is an underutilized modality of treatment. Because group life is crucial to adolescent development, group psychotherapy remains a treatment of choice for adolescents. The poor social skills, cognitive distortions, deficient coping patterns, and pathological defenses exhibited by suicidal teenagers can be addressed in group therapy by providing a safe, cohesive group atmosphere, promoting a sense of universalization, exploring new coping and behavior patterns, and lending support.

Clearly, with the rise of suicidality as a presenting problem in many outpatient clinics in conjunction with budget and staff cuts, group therapy presents a practical, cost-effective treatment method. As Trautman and Shaffer (1984) have pointed out, there is a need for further research into treatment methodology, using operationally defined therapies, well-defined patient populations, and sensitive measures of change. It is hoped that group therapy of suicidal adolescents will be included in research and studies so that its efficacy and therapeutic potential can be further improved. We believe that group therapy for suicidal adolescents offers a medium of safety, support, and therapeutic benefit. We hope that in the future, more clinics and agencies will consider this method of treatment and thus create more of what Farberow (1972) has called a vital element in suicide prevention, "communities of concern."

REFERENCES

Asimos, C., & Rosen, D. (1978). Group treatment of suicidal and depressed persons: Indications for an open-ended group therapy program. *Bulletin of the Menninger Clinic, 42*(6), 515–518.

Billings, J., Rosen, D., Asimos, C., & Motto, J. (1974). Observations on long-term group therapy with suicidal and depressed persons. *Life-Threatening Behavior, 4*(3), 160–170.

Blos, P. (1967). The second individuation process of adolescence. *Psychoanalytic Study of the Child, 22,* 162–186.

Brent, D., Kalas, R., Edelbrock, C., Costello, A., Dulcan, M., & Conover, N. (1986). Psychopathology and its relationship to suicidal ideation in childhood and adolescence. *Journal of the American Academy of Child and Adolescent Psychiatry, 25*(5), 663–673.

Brent, D., Perper, J., Goldstein, C., Kolko, D., Allan, M., Allman, C., & Zelenak, J. (1988). Risk factors for adolescent suicide. *Archives of General Psychiatry, 45*(6), 581–588.

Davis, F., & Lohr, N. (1971). Special problems with the use of cotherapists in group psychotherapy. *International Journal of Group Psychotherapy, 21*(2), 943–958.

Farberow, N. (1972). Vital process in suicide prevention: Group psychotherapy as a community of concern. *Life-Threatening Behavior, 2*(4), 239–251.

Farberow, N., & Schneidman, E. (1961). The suicide prevention center. In N. Farberow & E. Schneidman, (Eds.), *The cry for help* (pp. 3–19). New York: McGraw-Hill.

Garland, A., Shaffer K., & Whittle, B. (1989). A national survey of school-based, adolescent suicide prevention programs. *Journal of the American Academy of Child and Adolescent Psychiatry, 28*(6), 931–934.

Garland, J., Jones, H., & Kolodny, R. (1973). A model for stages in development in social work groups. In S. Bernstein (Ed.), *Explorations in group work: Essays in theory and practice* (pp. 21–30). Boston: Milford House.

Grunebaum, H., & Solomon, L. (1982). Toward a theory of peer relationships: On the stages of social development and their relationship to group psychotherapy. *International Journal of Group Psychotherapy, 32*(3), 283–307.

Hackel, J., & Asimos, C. (1981). Resistances encountered in starting a group therapy program for suicide attempters in varied administrative settings. *Suicide and Life-Threatening Behavior, 11*(2), 93–98.

Motto, J. (1990). Group psychotherapy of suicidal adolescents. In M. Seligman & L. Marshak (Eds.), *Group psychotherapy: Interventions with special populations* (pp. 164–173). Boston: Allyn-Bacon.

Pfeffer, C. R. (1986). *The suicidal child.* New York: The Guilford Press.

Ross, C., & Motto, J. (1984). Group counseling for suicidal adolescents. In H. Sudak, A. Ford, & N. Rushforth (Eds.), *Suicide in the young* (pp. 367–392). Boston: John Wright-PSG.

Scheidlinger, S. (1974). On the concept of the "mother group." *International Journal of Group Psychotherapy, 24*(4), 417–428.

Scheidlinger, S. (1985). Group treatment of adolescents: An overview. *American Journal of Orthopsychiatry, 55*(1), 102–111.

Scheidlinger, S., & Aronson, S. (1991). Group psychotherapy of adolescents. In M. Slomowitz (Ed.), *Adolescent psychotherapy* (pp. 103–119). Washington, DC: American Psychiatric Press.

Scheidlinger, S., & Porter, K. (1980). Group therapy combined with individual psychotherapy. In T. Karasu & L. Bellak (Eds.), *Specialized techniques in individual psychotherapy* (pp. 426–440). New York: Brunner/Mazel.

Shaffer, D., Garland, A., Gould, M., Fisher, P., & Trautman, P. (1988). Preventing teen suicide: A critical review. *Journal of the American Academy of Child and Adolescent Psychiatry, 27*(6), 675–687.

Shaffer, D., Garland, A., Vieland, V., Underwood, M., & Busner, C. (1991). The impact of curriculum-based suicide prevention programs for teenagers. *Journal of the American Academy of Child and Adolescent Psychiatry, 30*(4), 588–596.

Slavson, S. R. (1950). *Analytic group psychotherapy.* New York: Columbia University Press.

Trautman, P., & Shaffer, D. (1984). Treatment of child and adolescent suicide attempters. In H. Sudak, A. Ford, & N. Rushforth (Eds.), *Suicide in the young* (pp. 307–322). Boston: John Wright-PSG.

Yalom, I. (1975). *The theory and practice of group psychotherapy.* New York: Basic Books.

11

Suicide Attempts in Puerto Rican Adolescent Females
A Sociocultural Perspective and Family Treatment Approach

LUIS H. ZAYAS AND
LAWRENCE A. DYCHE

To understand the ethnic and cultural issues that clinicians face in the treatment of inner-city Latina* adolescents following a suicide attempt, this chapter focuses on mainland Puerto Rican females with an emphasis on treating the adolescent and her family. We review common risk factors that Puerto Rican adolescents share with other non-Latino youth and discuss contextual risk factors that are unique to Puerto Rican and other Hispanic adolescents. From the discussion of contextual factors, we focus on the sociocultural and family situations of Puerto Rican adolescent females that influence suicide attempts and that can inform their treatment. Several case vignettes are included to illustrate points made in our discussion.

Like many of our colleagues who toil in urban hospitals serving Latino communities, we have been struck by the high frequency of suicide attempts in the biographies of adolescent Latinas. It may be these attempts that brought them to the attention of the mental health system, or previous suicide attempts may be reported in the course of medical or psychotherapeutic interventions for other presenting

---

*Inasmuch as there is no universally accepted term to refer to the same population group, we will use the terms "Latino" and "Hispanic" interchangeably in this chapter. Where we refer to specific literature, we have retained "Hispanic," "Latino," or another term as used by the authors of the original source.

problems. Suicidal behavior is often present in other family members also, frequently mothers and grandmothers. Still another startling feature is the similarity in these suicide attempts. Most commonly, we find escalating tensions between the adolescent and her parents that lead to an impulsive act during prolonged, stressful family crises. The attempt is frequently made by the ingestion of a pre-scribed or over-the-counter medication. An explicit desire to die is often absent; instead, the adolescent senses no other outlet for appar-ently insoluble problems (Zimmerman, 1991; Zimmerman & Zayas, in press).

Our experience has taught us that there are several social, cultural, and psychological factors that are unique to Hispanics and, in the case of this chapter, to Puerto Rican teenage girls. These factors seem to influence the tensions that mount in the family and ultimately lead to the suicide attempt. Before entering into this discussion, a compara-tive review of suicidal risks among Hispanic adolescents and other youth will help to highlight the specific sociocultural factors we posit as significant in the suicide attempt and in treatment.

Although accurate statistics on the frequency of suicide attempts and hospitalizations are not available, some estimates suggest that in 1988 alone, 15,458 suicide attempts by 10- to 19-year-olds were brought to the attention of the medical system (Holinger, 1990). Harkavy Freidman, Asnis, Boeck, and DiFiore (1987) report that in a population of 380 white, black, Hispanic, and Asian stu-dents in an urban high school, 53 percent of the adolescents had thought about killing themselves and 8.7 percent had tried to kill themselves at least once. More girls than boys reported having tried to kill themselves.

As members of the second largest Hispanic group in the United States and the largest in the Northeast, Puerto Rican adolescents are seen frequently in the emergency rooms of urban hospitals for suicidal behavior. (See Razin et al., 1991; Zayas, 1987.) In their sample, Razin and his colleagues note that Hispanic adolescents, especially females, accounted for over 25 percent of all patients admitted for suicidal be-havior, while accounting for only 1.4 percent of the population served by the hospital. Older data presented by Teicher (1970) suggest that Puerto Rican youth in New York City have higher rates of suicide at-tempts than do African-American and white youth.

COMPARATIVE RISK FACTORS FOR HISPANIC AND NON-HISPANIC YOUTH

Most of what we know about suicidality in Hispanic youth comes from the literature dealing with completed suicides. Smith, Mercy, and Warren (1985) found that, in five southwestern states, suicide among Hispanics tended to be a youthful phenomenon; 32.9 percent of all Hispanics who committed suicide were under the age of 25, compared to 17.3 percent of whites in the same age group. Similar results are reported by McIntosh (1987) in a study of ten states with Hispanic populations. However, Hispanic suicide rates are typically lower than those of whites overall. Wyche and Rotheram-Borus (1990) point out that Native American adolescents have the highest rate of completed suicides when compared with African- and Hispanic-American youth, who have among the lowest rates. Note that these data are on completed suicides; the demographic data on suicide attempters are inadequate for making accurate comparisons between youth of differing ethnocultural and racial backgrounds.

Nevertheless, a comparative view of suicidal youth can illustrate some of the similarities and differences between Hispanic and non-Hispanic adolescents. For the purpose of this chapter, we consider risk factors to be of two kinds: *common risk factors,* that is, shared characteristics among most youth; and *contextual risk factors,* that is, specific factors derived from the unique sociocultural milieus of ethnic-racial minority adolescents. In this chapter, we focus on the contextual risk factors of teenage Puerto Rican girls, although some factors can be generalized to other adolescent Latinas.

Common Risk Factors

In general, Puerto Rican adolescents, like other Hispanic adolescents, share many of the same psychosocial risk factors discussed in the empirical literature on adolescent suicidality in the general population. (See Chapter 2.) Any inventory of common risks in adolescent suicidal behavior would list such factors as chronic or acute depression; poor interpersonal problem-solving skills; low self-esteem; hopelessness; impulsivity and poor judgment; a history of physical and/or sexual abuse, whether by family members or others; family discord and disruption, including domestic violence and parental separation and divorce; major psychiatric illness in or substance abuse by one or both parents; the absence of a support network for the adolescent or her family; and impaired parent-adolescent relations (Chabrol & Moron, 1988; Husain, 1990; Motto, Heilbron, & Juster, 1985; Pfeffer, 1989; Plutchik & van Praag, 1990; Rich, Young, & Fowler, 1986; Slaby & MacGuire, 1989; Spirito, Brown, Overholser, & Fritz, 1989). In the following vignette, the parents' marital discord, father's alcohol abuse, and the increased responsibility for the care of a sibling were among the risk factors that are often shared by suicidal Hispanic and other non-Hispanic youths.

Case Example

At 16, Margarita had complained of her parents' "emotional separation" despite having an intact family. Although her father worked and provided for the family, he would stay out late at night to return home after the family was asleep. Her mother would take care of her husband's basic needs such as cooking, cleaning, and preparing his clothes, but there was no affection between them and very little communication. Margarita felt caught between her parents, taking care of her younger brother, age nine, so as to relieve her depressed mother. Margarita's parents bickered constantly, did not sleep together, did not share in household or child-related decisions, and did not engage in any family rituals that would keep the family cohesive. Her father's drinking escalated while her mother's depression deepened. Loving both parents yet feeling that neither of them listened to her pleas that they work out their differences and adequately parent their children, Margarita ingested more than a dozen Motrin (ibuprofen), necessitating medical hospitalization.

Psychiatric impairment in the adolescent or in a parent is common among both minority and nonminority suicidal adolescents.

Case Example

Rosa was 14 at the time she was admitted to the adolescent psychiatric unit following a serious suicide attempt (slashing her wrists). Rosa's attempt followed an episode of a homosexual encounter with an older woman in her building. This encounter was later discovered by her mother and extended family, who then berated Rosa, calling her "sick" and "stupid." The psychiatric evaluation suggested that Rosa was beginning to show features of a borderline personality organization. There was a history of promiscuous behavior, impulsivity, some drug use, truancy, and numerous incomplete treatment efforts. The family history also disclosed maternal promiscuity, alcoholism, and violence against other women. After six weeks in an evaluation service, residential treatment was recommended and accepted but then aborted three months later. Less than a year later, Rosa was killed in an automobile accident when joy-riding in a stolen car with friends.

Contextual Risk Factors

Contextual risk factors are the specific social and cultural experiences that are the architects of psychological responses to crises among different ethnocultural groups. In the case of Puerto Rican and other Hispanic teens, unique sociocultural and family variables impinge on the adolescent that may be different or less evident in non-Hispanic and non-immigrant youth. For Puerto Rican and Dominican youth, these include: (1) migration and consequent network dislocation; (2) glaring discrepancies between the old and the new cultures; (3) acculturation to the mainland culture; (4) importance of generational status in the mainland culture (first, second, or later generation); (5) traditional Hispanic family processes that guard certain cultural values that may be at odds with the majority culture; and (6) low socioeconomic status (Zayas, 1987; Zimmerman & Zayas, in press). The cases of Blanca and Gricel exemplify the influence of sociocultural factors on the suicide attempt.

Case Example

Blanca, a slender 14-year-old Puerto Rican girl with a quick smile, was brought to the pediatric clinic by her mother, who pulled the physician aside, pleading in broken English for assurance that her daughter was still a virgin. Perplexed by the request, the pediatrician explained that he could only examine the girl for signs of illness. When he saw Blanca alone, she broke into tears, complaining that her mother did not want her to be with boys, much less have sex. Blanca had to live two lives to fit in with her peers and still keep her mother satisfied. She told the doctor that she frequently thought that the only solution was to kill herself if this continued. On at least one occasion she had taken an excessive dose of aspirin so she could "forget everything and put it behind me," but the only result was severe intestinal cramps and vomiting.

In the case of Blanca, her mother's adherence to traditional cultural expectations with respect to her daughter's honor and the resulting distrust of the girl were the most notable influences in the suicide attempt. In the case of Gricel that follows, her mother's isolation, which stemmed from her migration and lack of English fluency, led to over-involvement with and overreliance on her daughter.

Case Example

Mrs. M brought 17-year-old Gricel to the emergency room one weekday evening after Gricel had drowsily confessed to her mother that she had taken a handful of her mother's Xanax because she wanted to die. Mrs. M told the emergency room staff that she was horrified and could not imagine what caused her daughter to do this. To the ER psychiatrist and social worker, Gricel presented as a shy, depressed, slightly obese girl who had always been a good student and seemed devoted to her mother. However, she complained that lately her mother would not let her out of her sight and seemed excessively demanding of Gricel's constant companionship. In the family history, it was learned that Mrs. M herself was 17 and pregnant when she left Santurce, Puerto Rico, and came to New York against her own mother's wishes. Finding New York a "lonely city," Mrs. M took refuge in her daughter's love, and Gricel grew to be her best friend, confidante, and translator of language and culture. Even though she knew her daughter was growing, she could not imagine a life without her. As Gricel matured and neared the end of high school, Mrs. M felt more fearful of the impending loss of her daughter to college and the world. For the last month, she had told Gricel that the girl's disrespectful attitude was giving her a nervous breakdown and that the doctor had to give her tranquilizers. The night of the overdose, Gricel wanted to tell her mother that she was suffering too.

In the case of Migdalia, a combination of an older, parentified sibling and traditional cultural expectations about a girl's role and behaviors led to the suicide attempt.

Case Example

Migdalia, 15, was the second of four children. Her older brother, Pablo, at 17, had assumed the paternal role with his mother's explicit support since the death of their father two years before. The younger siblings, 11 and 9, were often Migdalia's responsibility while Mother worked. While Migdalia had complained at home loudly about her brother's rigidity and abuse of power, her mother would settle the difference by mildly reprimanding Pablo about his overuse of power with Migdalia. Migdalia resented her mother's failure to take her complaints about her brother's behavior seriously. On the afternoon of her suicide attempt, Migdalia had been playing with friends in a video arcade that also housed a pool hall generally frequented by some older men. When Pablo discovered her there by coincidence, he launched into a loud reprimand heard by Migdalia's peers and adults nearby that she had disobeyed her family's rules, that only a tramp would be seen in a place where men played pool, smoked, and drank alcohol, and that she had shamed herself and her family. In view of peers, neighbors, and strangers, he forcibly pulled her from the arcade and held her roughly by the elbow until they reached their apartment. Shortly after, Migdalia created a "cocktail" from different prescribed and over-the-counter medications. Pablo discovered her in her room pale and disoriented and took her to a local hospital where she was then hospitalized. Migdalia complained to the consultation-liaison psychologist that she could think of no other way of getting her brother and mother to listen to her needs. She longed for her dead father who would have disapproved of the pool hall but "would never have embarrassed and humiliated me the way my brother did."

SOCIOCULTURAL FACTORS AND
TREATMENT IMPLICATIONS

We see family intervention as the most effective modality with Puerto Rican and other Hispanic adolescents. Among the contextual factors described here, three—the migration experience, the dynamics of acculturation, and intergenerational family processes—are especially germane to family treatment. We discuss each factor in turn and outline implications for treatment.

Migration
We believe that the stress which migration poses for the Puerto Rican family is significant and can become focused with particular intensity on the adolescent female. As a precursor of acculturation, migration should be thought of as a crisis-inducing process, in spite of the family's desire to move. Geographic relocation, even within the same culture, fragments social support systems and removes the individual from

the orienting effects provided by a familiar sense of place. Within most immigrant Hispanic families, the rearing and socialization of children rest heavily on the mother, who works in concert with a tightly knit female support system that extends vertically to grandmothers and aunts and horizontally to female siblings, cousins, and friends. When migration severs these bonds, the mother is left without critically needed resources. Our experience has shown that when these women begin to negotiate their maternal roles in the absence of supportive females, they often turn within the nuclear family for assistance. Typically, they rely on an oldest daughter and create a bond with her that, while temporarily functional, sets the stage for severe problems with the daughter's adolescent individuation.

Acculturation

Acculturation is the process of adapting to the rules, roles, and expectations of the new culture. It involves matters as diverse as language, dress, and manners. Because it can cause people to question their deepest assumptions and challenge their most fixed habits, it is inevitably a source of crisis at both the individual and family levels. Adults typically resist acculturation; they make essential adaptations to the new setting, but seek to create networks and communities that allow for the preservation of their native culture. Children, however, must face the new culture during their formative years, before their sense of self is consolidated; almost unavoidably, children learn both the culture of their family and of the host society. Culture prescribes a variety of matters critical to family functioning, including behavior between parents and children, gender roles, and sexual behavior. As children, Latina girls in the United States attempt to absorb the dramatically discrepant expectations of a traditional, family-oriented culture and one oriented to individualism and achievement. In adolescence, when the influence of the outside world on the Latina increases, she and her parents are faced with an extraordinarily demanding interpersonal situation. This situation requires that, to meet the challenge successfully, each of them makes significant adjustments in their relationship. Some Hispanic parents and their daughters manage the struggle productively with compromises and understanding. Other families fail, frequently leading to dysfunction and fragmentation.

Intergenerational Family Dynamics and Processes

Another dimension that plays an especially significant role in the suicide attempt is intergenerational family processes. When combined with the stress of migration and acculturation, some aspects of the Latino family process may predispose the adolescent to crisis and acting out through suicidal behavior.

Tradition-bound cultures such as that of Puerto Ricans often contain rigid role constraints on the female that place an intense burden on the interaction between adolescent daughter and parents. Traditional gender role socialization for the female is typified by some degree of restrictiveness, especially regarding sexuality (as shown in the case vignettes of Blanca and Migdalia). This restrictiveness, at its extremes, is at odds with the adolescent's developmental needs and the demands of the urban mainland sociocultural system that she must negotiate in school, at work, and with peers.

Traditionally oriented Puerto Rican families value a distinct hierarchy in their family relations. It is essential that the therapist recognize this preference for hierarchy in order to gain entry into the family system. Since the therapist represents an "expert" to the family, he or she will be ascribed a certain level of authority. This should be accepted graciously in order to facilitate engagement and gain leverage for influencing the family (Zayas & Bryant, 1984). Our clinical experience has taught us over the years that when the Puerto Rican family is in crisis, such as is reflected in the adolescent's emotional distress and behavioral problems (i.e., the suicide attempt or other acting-out disorder), it is often due to a disruption in the family's traditional organization and hierarchy. Among the most common and disturbing breakdowns in the migrant family's pattern of interacting occur when there is a sense of rupture in the mother-daughter relationship. (For a full discussion of this rupture and its repair, see Zimmerman, 1991, and Zimmerman and Zayas, in press.)

Research on Hispanic families has affirmed what clinicians and other observers have noted for years: Children of immigrants who either are born in the United States or arrive at an early age acculturate more rapidly than do their parents (Szapocznik, Scopetta, Kurtines, & Aranalde, 1978). More than simply learning English and losing some degree of fluency in their original Spanish, the child's acculturation frequently is accompanied by the adoption of a new set of values, attitudes, and behaviors, many of which are incompatible with the parents' original culture and their own socialization.

Much of acculturation is compounded by the natural developmental processes of both the family and adolescent. Life-stage transitions in a family demand flexibility. In Puerto Rican and other Hispanic families, these transitions, especially with the child in early and middle adolescence, are complicated when the adolescent "develops attachments to conflicting cultural values and behaviors" (Rio, Santiesteban, & Szapocznik, 1990, p. 212). This is especially important in Hispanic family functioning, since premigration intergenerational differences are dramatically heightened by discrepant rates of acculturation among migrant family members (Rio et al., 1990; Zimmerman & Zayas, in press).

How value differences between first- and second-generation Puerto Rican adolescent females and their parents are resolved are determined by the family's transactional patterns (Canino, 1982). Flexibility is essential in the family's capacity to deal effectively with the stress of migration and acculturation. Well-functioning, traditionally oriented Puerto Rican parents may appear initially to outsiders (e. g., interviewers, therapists) as unduly strict and interfering with their daughters, dominating conversations while the girls sit quietly and respectfully (Canino, 1982). Gradually, children are allowed to express ideas that are different from those of their parents, usually as parents engage with interviewers or therapists. In these families, traditional Puerto Rican values can coexist with newer values. Highly acculturated adolescent females who come from flexible, supportive, and adaptive families often do not embrace drastically different values from those of their parents (Canino, 1982). Instead, the adolescents manifest a balance between "behavioral acculturation" and "values acculturation." That is, the girls adopt changes in their behaviors—such as in dress, music and language choices, and foods—while holding to values and attitudes similar to those of their parents. This is especially true in relation to sexuality and family. By diminishing the disparity in acculturation between themselves and their parents, the girls avoid intergenerational stresses (Canino, 1982). Parents and adolescents use social support systems to help them disengage from one another without undue guilt and resentment (Zimmerman & Zayas, in press).

Dysfunctional families tolerate less self-differentiation. Family boundaries are less permeable, and there may be parental overinvolvement with the adolescent; these are important factors in our perspective on the suicidal adolescent, as shown in the case of Gricel. Triangulation occurs when intergenerational conflicts (especially, grandmother-mother-daughter) are apparent (Canino, 1982). Problematic families tend to be inflexible regarding the demands they face with a maturing adolescent and the attendant life-cycle changes the family must make.

In families of suicidal female adolescents, parents often remain rigid in their sex-role expectations and discourage role differentiation in the family. As our experience has shown, parents often are socially isolated from the community and the vast support system that they may have enjoyed in Puerto Rico. This is especially so for the mother, who often could turn to a network of sisters, female cousins and neighbors, and *madrinas* and *comadres* (godmothers and comothers) on the island but is now bereft of this natural support.

To integrate the sociocultural influences we have discussed here with a family-centered treatment approach, we conclude with a full case study.

Case Example

Sixteen-year-old Maritza was hospitalized on a medical ward following an overdose of her mother's iron tablets. The suicide attempt had followed an argument with her mother over a boyfriend, and replicated a suicide gesture two years before that resulted in a family treatment effort that was brief and unsatisfactory. The therapist met mother and daughter on the ward, explained the family work that would begin during hospitalization and continue after discharge, and showed them the outpatient clinic area. Both acknowledged need for help in "communicating," and an appointment was scheduled for three days after Maritza's discharge.

Maritza's mother, Mrs. C, came alone to the first appointment with a feeble excuse for her daughter's absence, and she seemed to welcome the therapist's agreement to see her individually. She poured out a sense of desperation and rage at her daughter's behavior and shared a fear that she might lose control with the girl and become violent. With the therapist's help, she described her own life and explained the complexities of her relationship with this daughter.

Mrs. C was her mother's third daughter and was born shortly after the family's migration from Fajardo, Puerto Rico. Soon after the move, her mother began to exhibit a pattern of depression and suicidality that resulted in several hospitalizations over her lifetime. Mrs. C came to be known as the "tough one" among her siblings, and she became pregnant with Maritza at age 15. When she returned from the hospital with her newborn, Mrs. C's mother assumed absolute control over the infant's care. After several months of struggle over who would care for the baby, Mrs. C relented. She then moved away from home, married, and bore two more daughters. She and her mother maintained tense but polite relations, and over the years Maritza treated Mrs. C as aunt rather than mother.

When Maritza was 13 she pressed to move back with her mother. Several months of negotiation accomplished this, though it was over her grandmother's protests and threats of suicide. Her grandmother told Maritza that her room would be kept waiting, implying that her reunion with mother would certainly fail. Mrs. C was gratified by Maritza's decision, but as her daughter settled into the family, she found inheriting a teenager more complicated then expected. Maritza had grown accustomed to being the "baby" at her grandmother's home, and showed little patience with her younger sisters. In the year preceding the suicide attempt, tensions had been building and tempers flaring, with Maritza's willful stubbornness the flash point of her mother's anger.

The following week, when Maritza came to the therapy session with her mother, the tension between them was palpable. It quickly became apparent to the therapist that discussion of the suicide attempt in such an atmosphere could only inflame their mutual anger and disappointment. He opted instead, with a large genogram as a backdrop, to draw out whatever themes could link them. Their mutual enjoyment of food provided a medium through which to tell the story of their family, and changes in food preferences and diet symbolized the process of acculturation. From the story of Mrs. C's learning to cook came a recounting of her intense struggle around leaving home when she was Maritza's age.

The therapist addressed Maritza, saying that last week he learned that her mother had also been quite an independent person as a teenager. Maritza, intrigued with hearing her mother's story, smiled thoughtfully. He asked Mrs. C if she ever noticed how deeply her daughter admired her independent side. "Admired?" Mrs. C repeated, looking stunned for a moment. Then she smiled. "I guess so. I had to be strong." The therapist affirmed that "you had to be strong to finally bring your family together." Only with this sense of connection established did the therapist refer back to the suicide attempt and their fear of discussing it. He emphasized the complexity of their family story and that time would be needed to make up for their many years apart.

A second joint session continued the examination of family history for positive themes and provided an opportunity for the therapist to meet one of Maritza's half sisters. Then, on the afternoon before the third session, the therapist received a call from Mrs. C. With frightened desperation she recounted how Maritza, in a rage at her boyfriend, had cut up the stuffed animals he had given her. Maritza had just left to deliver the pieces to him. Mrs. C indicated that her "instinct" was to follow Maritza since she feared violence between Maritza and her boyfriend. However, she knew that in her past attempts to intervene when Maritza fought with her boyfriend, she found herself having to wrestle Maritza out of the boyfriend's apartment, causing anger between Maritza and herself.

Sensing the dramatized quality of these episodes, the therapist counseled Mrs. C to wait at home for a call from Maritza or the boyfriend's mother. He gave her an emergency number to reach him. The following day, Mrs. C came to the session triumphant and recounted that Maritza had returned unhurt a few hours after the conversation with the therapist. Though Maritza remained aloof during the session, she was positively connected to the therapy process. From this point on, the therapy began to emphasize structural themes, and in the fourth session Maritza shared her suicidal feelings in some detail with a new sense of safety resulting from improved communication with her mother.

The treatment extended to 11 sessions over five months. In several of the latter sessions, Mrs. C came without Maritza. She was seen once with her husband and twice with a woman friend. (The husband had to this point refused participation in the sessions since he felt that the problem was between Mrs. C and her daughter; the friend provided much-needed support to Mrs. C as a confidante.) Her relationships with her family of origin were explored and her aspirations to resume work discussed. A follow-up six months after the end of treatment showed that Maritza's behavior had continued to be manageable and her school performance improved. Mrs. C and her friend both began work as teacher's aides.

This case reflects several of the issues discussed earlier in families of suicidal teenage Puerto Rican girls and a family-directed treatment approach. In part, Mrs. C and Maritza's drama was playing out the maternal grandmother's prophecy that Maritza would return in failure from her mother's home. Since clinical experience had shown that disparities in cultural values and acculturation, and parent-child separations caused by migration, were frequent elements in suicide attempts by teenage Latinas, the therapist helped focus Mrs. C and Maritza on each other and their experiences. The initial emphasis in therapy was to narrow the breach between Mrs. C and Maritza by including tension-reducing discussions of genograms, family history, and food.

Similarly, as was the case with Mrs. C and Maritza, clinical experience had pointed to problems in the establishment of boundaries between suicidal Latina adolescents and their mothers. Mrs. C's overinvolvement with Maritza was dealt with effectively in the therapy through two means. First of all, the therapist provided directive intervention on how Mrs. C could disengage from her daughter's relationship to the boyfriend when the young lovers quarreled. This technique was based on a trusting relationship with the therapist that offered support in the absence of support from her husband. The approach also helped Maritza differentiate more from and rely less on her mother to intervene in her life in ways that served only to fuel their tension.

A second way the therapist helped to diminish Mrs. C's involvement with Maritza was by his tacit acceptance of the female friend's presence in the sessions, thereby supporting Mrs. C's attachment to a helpful adult female, which experience she lacked in her extended family. Encouraging Mrs. C to enter the labor force was intended to help lessen her social isolation, improve her own self-esteem, and model for Maritza a new role.

CONCLUSION

This chapter has reviewed the common and contextual risk factors that influence suicide attempts among mainland adolescent Puerto Rican girls. In particular, we have explored how the processes of migration and acculturation interact with family organization and adolescent development. Based on our clinical experience and informed by research findings, we have emphasized a family-centered treatment approach, demonstrated in the final case example.

REFERENCES

Canino, G. (1982). Transactional family patterns: A preliminary exploration of Puerto Rican female adolescents. In R. E. Zambrana (Ed.), *Work, family, and health: Latina women in transition* (Monograph No. 7, pp. 27–36). New York: Hispanic Research Center, Fordham University.

Chabrol, H., & Moron, P. (1988). Depressive disorders in 100 adolescents who attempted suicide. *American Journal of Psychiatry, 145*(3), 379.

Harkavy Friedman, J. M., Asnis, G. M., Boeck, M., & DiFiore, J. (1987). Prevalence of specific suicidal behaviors in a high school sample. *American Journal of Psychiatry, 144,* 1203–1206.

Holinger, P. (1990). The causes, impact, and preventability of childhood injuries in the United States: Childhood suicide in the United States. *American Journal of Diseases of Children, 144,* 670–676.

Husain, S. A. (1990). Current perspectives on the role of psychosocial factors in adolescent suicide. *Psychiatric Annals, 20*(3), 122–127.

McIntosh, J. L. (1987, May). *Hispanic suicide in ten U.S. states.* Paper presented at the joint meeting of the American Association of Suicidology and International Association for Suicide Prevention, San Francisco, CA.

Motto, J. A., Heilborn, D. C., & Juster, R. P. (1985). Development of a clinical instrument to estimate suicide risk. *American Journal of Psychiatry, 142,* 1061–1064.

Pfeffer, C. R. (Ed.) (1989). *Suicide among youth: Perspectives on risk and prevention.* Washington, DC: American Psychiatric Press.

Plutchik, R., & van Praag, H. M. (1990). Psychosocial correlates of suicide and violence risk. In H. M. van Praag, R. Plutchik, & A. Apter (Eds.), *Violence and suicidality: Perspectives in clinical and psychobiological research* (pp. 37–65). New York: Brunner/Mazel.

Razin, A. M., O'Dowd, M. A., Nathan, A., Rodriguez, I., Goldfield, A., Martin, C., Goulet, L., Scheftel, S., Mezan, P., & Mosca, J. (1991). Suicidal behavior among inner-city Hispanic adolescent females. *General Hospital Psychiatry, 13,* 45–58.

Rich, C. L., Young, D., & Fowler, R. C. (1986). San Diego suicide study: I. Young vs. old subjects. *Journal of Comparative and Physiological Psychology, 58,* 187–193.

Rio, A., Santiesteban, D. A., & Szapocznik, J. (1990). Treatment approaches for Hispanic drug-abusing adolescents. In R. Glick & J. Moore (Eds.), *Drugs in Hispanic communities* (pp. 203–229). New Brunswick, NJ: Rutgers University Press.

Slaby, A. E., & MacGuire, P. L. (1989). Residential management of suicidal adolescents. *Residential Treatment for Children and Youth, 7*(1), 23–43.

Smith, J. C., Mercy, J. A., & Warren, C. W. (1985). Comparison of suicides among Anglos and Hispanics in five southwestern states. *Suicide and Life-Threatening Behavior, 15,* 14–26.

Spirito, A., Brown, L., Overholser, J., & Fritz, G. (1989). Attempted suicide in adolescence: A review and critique of the literature. *Clinical Psychology Review, 9*(3), 335–363.

Szapocznik, J., Scopetta, M. A., Kurtines, W., & Aranalde, M. A. (1978). Theory and measurement of acculturation. *Inter-American Journal of Psychology, 12,* 113–130.

Teicher, J. D. (1970). Children and adolescents who attempt suicide. *Pediatric Clinics of North America, 17,* 685–696.

Wyche, K. F., & Rotheram-Borus, M. J. (1990). Suicidal behavior among minority youth in the United States. In A. R. Stiffman & L. E. Davis (Eds.), *Ethnic issues in adolescent mental health* (pp. 323–338). Newbury Park, CA: Sage.

Zayas, L. H. (1987). Toward an understanding of suicide risks in young Hispanic females. *Journal of Adolescent Research, 2*(1), 1–11.

Zayas, L. H. (1989). A retrospective on "The Suicidal Fit" in mainland Puerto Ricans: Research issues. *Hispanic Journal of Behavioral Sciences, 11*(1), 46–57.

Zayas, L. H., & Bryant, C. (1984). Culturally sensitive treatment of adolescent Puerto Rican girls and their families. *Child and Adolescent Social Work Journal, 1,* 235–253.

Zimmerman, J. K. (1991). Crossing the desert alone: An etiological model of female adolescent suicidality. In C. Gilligan, A. G. Rogers, & D. L. Tolman (Eds.), *Women, girls, and psychotherapy: Reframing resistance* (pp. 223–240). New York: Haworth Press.

Zimmerman, J. K., & Zayas, L. H. (in press). Suicidal adolescent Latinas: Culture, female development, and restoring the mother-daughter relationship. In S. S. Canetto & D. Lester (Eds.), *Women and suicide: A feminist perspective.* New York: Springer.

12

Adolescent Suicide
Diagnosis, Psychopharmacology, and Psychotherapeutic Management

JEFFREY P. KAHN,
KAREN J. PROWDA, AND
PAUL D. TRAUTMAN

Adolescent suicide is a significant public health concern and is the focus of increasing attention in the psychiatric literature. Many studies examine risk factors, demographics, and psychotherapeutic interventions in the suicide-prone adolescent (e.g., Shaffer, Garland, Gould, Fisher, & Trautman, 1988). The large majority of adolescent suicide victims and suicide attempters have diagnosable psychiatric disorders, and recent studies have begun to examine specific psychopathology (e.g., Brent et al., 1993). Much work has focused on crisis intervention and community based efforts related to treating the suicidal adolescent (e.g., Leenaars & Wenckstern, 1991). In contrast, there are relatively few studies of appropriate medication strategies or of psychotherapeutic management of medication response.

In considering the relevant literature, it is important to keep certain caveats in mind. For example, there is an essential distinction between those teens with suicidal thoughts or suicidal gestures, sometimes termed "parasuicides," and those teens who show true suicidal behaviors and completed suicides. The complex determinants for each of these groups may well be different. Hirsch, Walsh, and Draper (1982) reviewed studies of treatment intervention in parasuicide and concluded that altering behavior or environment, prescribing then conventional antidepressant medications, and social and medical support do not lower substantially the recidivism rate. There also are practical difficulties in conducting medication trials in the smaller number of

219

adolescents who have survived bona fide suicide attempts and who may be difficult to locate or recruit into studies. Importantly, though, there is evidence that depression in adolescents, as in adults, is under-recognized and undertreated. Keller, Lavori, Beardslee, Wunder, and Ryan (1991) reported on 38 adolescents with a median age of 14 years who were diagnosed with major depression. Of this group, only 18 percent received any treatment for depression, and only one subject received pharmacologic treatment (a benzodiazepine).

Suicidal thought and behavior can be the end result of a variety of medication responsive syndromes. In treating this population, the clinician uses his or her expertise in combining accurate psychiatric diagnosis, appropriate pharmacologic management, and psychotherapy. The clinician must be skilled in diagnosing specific psychiatric syndromes in the adolescent population. Rather than a problem of teenage years alone, it has been suggested that the serious problem of adolescent suicide may represent the onset of ongoing adult emotional turmoil (Shaffer et al., 1988). While suicide rates start to increase substantially in teen years, they do not then disappear after adolescence. A peak in the 20s is followed by another in the elderly, especially in white males.

The potential to miss psychopathology in the adolescent may be increased by exclusive focus on issues of adolescent turmoil, family discord, and drug and alcohol abuse. Moreover, suicidal adolescents often are angry at or defiant of authority, and consequently can be uncooperative during both evaluation and treatment. It is therefore essential to establish a trusting therapeutic alliance with the suicidal adolescent as early as possible and to help him or her find value and personal meaning in the treatment process. Often it is helpful to specify to the adolescent the psychiatrist's role as physician rather than as an agent of parental authority. Additional history also should be obtained from family members. However, the severity of suicidal thought is obtained chiefly from the adolescent; parents often are unaware of and underreport this symptom (Brent et al., 1986; Zimmerman & Asnis, 1991). Clinical assessment always must take into account the possible relationship of suicidal thoughts, gestures, and attempts to specific and treatable psychiatric diagnoses. In the absence of proper diagnosis and medication management, psychiatric syndromes often will continue unabated and make proper psychotherapeutic management difficult or impossible.

SPECIFIC DIAGNOSTIC ENTITIES

In evaluating the suicidal adolescent, certain specific diagnostic entities should be considered for pharmacologic intervention. Since the literature on medication management in adolescents is limited, adult drug studies often are used in treatment decisions. Dosages used in adolescents may be similar to adults, but the youth's smaller physical size and sometimes higher rate of metabolism may influence drug levels and distribution. There may be a role for medication in the management of adolescents with affective illness, anxiety disorders, and schizophrenia and other psychoses. Drug and alcohol abuse and emerging character disorders, including borderline and antisocial personality disorders, also are commonly associated with some of these syndromes and with suicidal thoughts.

AFFECTIVE DISORDERS

This section considers the use of pharmacotherapy in suicidal adolescents with affective disorders, including major depression, dysthymia and atypical depression, and bipolar disorder.

Major Depression

Case 1

Celia was a 17-year-old twelfth grader who was referred by a social worker for symptoms of depression. She had lived with her parents in the United States for four years, having moved from another country because of better educational opportunities. Following the death of her older brother in military combat, she reported two months of deterioration of mood, often experiencing irritability, withdrawal from her family, self-reproach, crying spells, fatigue, and difficulty sustaining interest in activities she formerly enjoyed. She had middle insomnia and decreased appetite, often missing meals. Celia had thoughts of cutting her wrists as a form of self-punishment. Her parents noted new onset conduct problems including truancy, lying, stealing money from them, and staying out all night with friends. She was diagnosed with major depressive disorder and treated with fluoxetine 20 mg every other morning. Upon follow-up, she reported improved sleep, energy, and mood with an absence of suicidal thoughts.

Case 2

Shannon was a 17-year-old eleventh grader who reported a one-year history of depressive symptoms with no clear precipitant that included self-denigration, depressed mood, poor concentration, anhedonia, deterioration in grades, early insomnia, and preoccupation with thoughts that she'd be better off dead. Shannon superficially cut her wrists on several different occasions when feeling angry and upset. She was admitted to a psychiatric hospital when she felt unable to control urges to hurt herself. She was diagnosed with major depression and treated with desipramine for eight weeks. A serum desipramine level of 100 ng/ml was subtherapeutic. Attempts to increase desipramine levels were limited by QRS widening on the electrocardiogram. Desipramine was tapered and discontinued when her depressive symptoms continued unabated. Treatment with fluoxetine 20 mg every day was initiated. Despite initial improvements in motivation and energy, Shannon remained anxious, worried, and sad. An increase of fluoxetine to 40 mg per day then led to symptomatic remission.

Often precipitated by object loss and family turmoil, major depression is a biological and psychological disorder that is commonly associated with suicidal thought and action. Depression in youth is now recognized as a valid clinical syndrome. Kovacs, Feinberg, Crouse-Novak, Paulauskas, and Finkelstein (1984) characterized adjustment disorder with depressed mood, major depression, and dysthymia in children age eight to 13 years, noting that remission was most favorable for adjustment disorders and least so for dysthymia. The standardized *Diagnostic and Statistical Manual* (DSM-IV; American Psychiatric Association, 1994) criteria for major depression are widely adopted in child and adolescent studies. They require dysphoria or pervasive anhedonia for at least two weeks. In addition, four out of eight of the following features must be present for two weeks: appetite disturbance, sleep disturbance, motor agitation or retardation, anhedonia, loss of energy, self-reproach or guilt, impaired ability to concentrate, and recurrent thoughts of death or suicide. Further, depression in the adolescent may be manifest by behavioral changes including delinquency, risk-taking, aggression, violence, drug abuse, and sexual promiscuity (Rutter & Hersov, 1985). In fact, substance abuse often can be the most evident symptom of depression. (See

"Dysthymia and Atypical Depression" and "Bipolar Disorder" that follow.)

Studies have demonstrated the association between depression and adolescent suicide. Shaffer and associates (1988) noted that adolescent male and female suicides from a general population included 21 percent and 50 percent respectively diagnosed with major depression, compared with 2 percent diagnosed with major depression in normal adolescent control groups. Brent and coworkers (1988) noted that major depression was present, by parent history, in 62.5 percent of suicide attempters and 40.7 percent of completed suicides in children and adolescents ranging in age from six to 18 years. Trautman, Rotheram-Borus, Dopkins, and Lewin (1991) reported that depression was present in 42 percent of the suicide attempters in a sample of minority female girls aged 12 to 17 years. Myers and associates (1991) reported that among youths seven to 17 years old diagnosed with major depressive disorder, suicidal risk was predicted by the severity of depression and by the presence of conduct disorder and impulsivity. Pfeffer and colleagues (1991) reported, in a six- to eight-year follow-up study, that 4- to 14-year-old children who were recidivist suicide attempters were seven times more likely to have a mood disorder compared with those who had never attempted suicide.

Pharmacologic management of major depression in adolescents has been modeled on treatments of depressed adults. Few rigorous studies specifically assess the effectiveness of tricyclic antidepressants in the depressed adolescent. While the available data do not provide consistent evidence for the efficacy of tricyclics in treating depressed adolescents (Pfeffer, Peskin, & Siefker, 1992; Preskorn, Weller, & Weller, 1982; Puig-Antich et al., 1979; Puig-Antich et al., 1987; Ryan et al., 1986; Strober, Freeman, & Rigali, 1990), they may still prove useful for melancholic depression.

In treating depressed and suicidal adolescents, caution must be exercised in using tricyclic antidepressants and other medications that can be lethal in overdose. Cardiovascular side effects are of concern in all patients treated with tricyclic antidepressants, and can include postural hypotension, sinus tachycardia, prolonged intracardiac conduction times (as in Shannon's case), arrhythmias, direct myocardial depression, and such other electrocardiogram (ECG) changes as T-wave flattening or inversion. Young people may be more vulnerable to cardiotoxic effects than adults (Baldessarini, 1990). A baseline

ECG should be obtained prior to beginning a tricyclic antidepressant, repeated when dosage of tricyclic reaches 3 mg/kg/day, and then repeated again with every subsequent dosage increase. Of particular concern are evidence of cardiac conduction abnormalities such as PR interval exceeding 0.18 seconds, QRS interval greater than 130 percent of baseline, cardiac arrhythmia, tachycardia, or heart block.

There are at least four reported cases of sudden deaths in children taking desipramine, although a causal role has not yet been documented (Riddle et al., 1991). Routine monitoring of children on any tricyclic antidepressant should include serial ECGs and measurements of plasma drug concentration. Puig-Antich and associates (1987) found that total plasma concentrations of imipramine (imipramine plus desipramine) in depressed prepubertal children served as a better predictor of clinical response than dosage levels.

Fluoxetine is preferable to tricyclic antidepressants in certain clinical situations. One recent open study found that 64 percent of subjects ages 16 to 24 years with major depression who failed to respond to prior treatments with tricyclic antidepressants showed a therapeutic response to fluoxetine (Boulos, Kutcher, Gardner, & Young, 1992). McBride, Trautman, and Glick (unpublished data) looked at 17 subjects with major depressive disorder, including three with chronic dysthymia, who had failed to respond to psychotherapy alone. After eight weeks of fluoxetine treatment (20 to 40 mg daily), all were somewhat or much improved in depressive symptoms, and 15 of 17 were somewhat or much improved in psychosocial function. Importantly, since fluoxetine is far less toxic than tricyclic antidepressants in overdose, it is sometimes a more prudent choice for treatment of a depressed and suicidal adolescent. There are only two deaths reported from overdose of fluoxetine, and both occurred in combination with other drugs and/ or alcohol (*Physicians' Desk Reference,* 1994). Newer serotonin reuptake inhibitors, such as sertraline and paroxetine, may prove to have therapeutic benefits and safety that are similar to fluoxetine.

Dysthymia and Atypical Depression

Case 3

Mary was a 15-year-old ninth grader who presented for treatment after a suicide attempt by overdose. She reported a three-year history of feeling overly sensitive, burdened by her troubles, and easily saddened. She described long-standing difficulties getting along with her parents. Over the past year, in the context of continuing conflict with parents over curfews, Mary had developed anhedonia, daily crying spells, initial insomnia and early-morning awakening, substantial weight gain, and difficulties concentrating. These symptoms allowed diagnosis of dysthymic disorder with concurrent major depression, as well as parent-child conflict. She was treated in family therapy and with fluoxetine 20 mg every other day. Mary initially experienced improved mood and sleep, but ongoing family conflict contributed to some continuing distress. Importantly, family therapy was later aided by fluoxetine treatment of similar depressive symptoms in Mary's mother.

Case 4

Tom was a 17-year-old high school senior. For the past two years, he had had periods when he would feel tired, depressed, and lethargic for weeks at a time. Although he could feel cheerful with friends, he also felt himself more than usually sensitive to rejection and criticism. He had no symptoms of an anxiety disorder. Soon after his depression started, he found that heroin offered temporary alleviation of his symptoms. With increasing despondence about school, family, and his girlfriend, though, he took so much heroin one day that he lost consciousness. During medical and psychiatric hospitalization, he acknowledged his suicidal thoughts and later started outpatient treatment.

Dysthymia is another affective diagnosis to consider in the suicidal adolescent. Chronic symptoms are part of this syndrome, with one study showing a median duration of three and one-half years (Kovacs et al., 1984). The clinical presentation of adolescent dysthymia includes one-year duration of depressed or irritable mood accompanied by at least two of the following: poor appetite or overeating, insomnia or hypersomnia, low energy, low self-esteem, poor concentration or difficulties making decisions, and feelings of hopelessness. With its chronic symptoms, dysthymia often is less apparent initially to both child and parent than an acute major depression. Double depressions may occur as well, where major depression is superimposed on long-standing dysthymia. The literature on treating adult dysthymia includes many medications and suggests the particular efficacy of monamine oxidase inhibitors (MAOIs) and fluoxetine (Harrison & Stewart, 1993).

 Many dysthymic and other depressed patients also meet diagnositic criteria for atypical depression, which is newly referenced in DSM-IV (American Psychiatric Association, 1994). One study reports that about 25 percent of adult depressives suffer from atypical depression (Asnis, McGinn, & Sanderson, in press). Onset of atypical depression is typically in middle to late adolescence. Diagnostic criteria require mood reactivity in addition to at least two of the following symptoms: fatigue, hypersomnia (increased sleep), hyperphagia (weight gain), leaden paralysis (a leaden feeling in the arms or legs), and a pattern of heightened interpersonal rejection-sensitivity (as in Case 3). Both MAOIs (Quitkin et al., 1989) and fluoxetine (Pande, Haskett, & Graden, 1992) are effective treatments. MAOIs, though, are associated with more side effects, including potentially fatal hypertensive crises. A restrictive diet that prohibits such tyramine-containing foods as cheese, chocolate, and red wine is required when taking MAOIs. This can be problematic for teenagers who may routinely partake of pizza or candy. Furthermore, MAOIs in the hands of an adolescent who is impulsive or rebellious may pose a serious risk as a result of parental defiance, dietary noncompliance, or overdose.

Substance abuse often represents self-medication for underlying chronic anxiety or depressive symptoms in suicidal adolescents. (See Case 4 earlier and Case 5 that follows.) The underlying symptoms thus are easily masked or overlooked. Using a psychological autopsy approach to suicide victims ages 11 to 19 years, Strober and associates (1988) found that mood disorders were coexistent with either alcohol and drug abuse, conduct disorder or other mental disorders in 76 percent of victims and 24 percent of controls. Martunnen, Aro, Henriksson, and Lonnqvist (1991) reported on Finnish adolescent suicide victims, ages 13 to 19 years. One-third of them had a post-mortem diagnosis of coexistent alcohol abuse or dependence, and two-thirds of those were also depressed. Shaffi, Carrigan, Whittinghill, and Derrick (1985) reported that 70 percent of youths ages 12 to 19 years who had completed suicide had a history of drug or alcohol abuse. While drug abuse is not medication responsive per se, it commonly reflects underlying medication-responsive syndromes. With pharmacological treatment, the drug abuse itself then becomes more amenable to treatment, but it still often requires rehabilitation programs, self-help groups, and so on.

Bipolar Disorder

Case 5

Bruce was a 17-year-old male with a history of two prior suicide attempts and prior hospitalization for depression. That depression responded to a combination of imipramine, chlorpromazine, thyroid hormone, and dextroamphetamine, and he remained well for two months. Within two weeks of chlorpromazine discontinuation, however, he became increasingly irritable and argumentative. Using forged checks and money stolen from his mother, he bought hundreds of dollars' worth of new clothing. He abruptly stopped seeing his old friends and spent time instead with a drug-abusing crowd. Bruce soon began using marijuana daily, with frequent alcoholic binges. Four days before hospitalization, he became unconscious from alcohol and was seen briefly in an emergency room.

On the day of admission, he argued with his father, broke a table in his grandmother's house, made extravagant claims about his musical genius, threatened to throw his infant niece across a room, and said that he would find a gun to shoot himself. On a psychiatric inpatient unit, Bruce had pressured speech even while doing headstands on his bed. Despite his agitation and prior depression, all medications were stopped. Instead, treatment focused solely on diagnoses of substance abuse and personality disorder. Following continued agitation, irritability, and disruptive behavior, he was transferred to another hospital. Initiation of lithium 300 mg tid brought gradual remission of his symptoms. Except for occasional drinking bouts, Bruce remained well on lithium until a recurrent depression six years later.

Like unipolar depression, bipolar disorder once was thought to be rare in childhood and adolescence. However, studies of adults found that about one-fifth of adults with bipolar illness reported onset of symptoms before age 19 years (Carlson, Davenport, & Jamison, 1977). The clinical features of mania in adolescence are similar to those described in adults, including decreased need for sleep, irritability, excessive spending, hypersexuality, increased motor activity, flight of ideas, and psychotic ideation (including delusions of grandiosity or persecution). Suicidal thoughts may be masked as grandiose fantasies. For example, a suicide attempt during a manic episode might involve jumping from a window in order to fly, without any conscious suicidal intent.

Bipolar patients with onset in childhood or adolescence may have increased risk for both suicide and rapid cycling, as compared with patients who have a later age of onset (Olsen, 1961; Welner, Welner, & Fishman, 1979). More recently, Brent and colleagues (1988) compared adolescent suicide victims with suicidal inpatients ages 13 to 19 years and found that a diagnosis of bipolar disorder was significantly more prevalent among the suicide victims. Shaffer and associates (1988) reported that adolescents with bipolar psychosis constitute a group at probable high risk for suicide.

Treatment of manic depressive illness generally involves lithium in the acute manic episode and in long-term prophylaxis. DeLong and Aldershof (1987) reported that 66 percent of 59 children with bipolar disorder were treated successfully with lithium. Strober, Freeman, and Rigali (1990) conducted a naturalistic study of 37 adolescents, ages 13 to 17 years old, with bipolar I illness who had been stabilized on lithium. The relapse rate of bipolar illness was nearly three times higher in the noncompliant patients than in those who continued lithium prophylaxis.

The same precautions in treating an adult with lithium pertain to treating adolescents. Because of risk for toxicity, administration of lithium is largely contraindicated in individuals with significant renal or cardiovascular disease, severe dehydration, or hyponatremia. Since long-term lithium use may cause hypothyroidism, preexisting thyroid disease also can be a contraindication. Thyroid function studies should be performed before starting lithium and then at six-month intervals thereafter. Of further concern is treatment of sexually active females, since lithium administration during pregnancy is associated with Ebstein's anomaly and other fetal defects. Consequently, medical evaluation before starting lithium should include a complete blood count, serum electrolytes, renal function measures (including serum creatinine and urinalysis), thyroid function tests, a pregnancy test, and an electrocardiogram. Another major concern associated with lithium is its narrow therapeutic window. Target serum lithium levels during acute mania are between 1 and 1.5 mEq/liter, while maintenance levels usually range between 0.6 and 1.2 mEq/liter. Regular blood tests should be done to monitor serum levels and to adjust lithium dose. As with tricyclic antidepressants, the potentially fatal consequences of lithium overdose are of great concern when administered to a suicidal adolescent. Carbamazepine is a useful alternative for treating lithium-resistant bipolar illness in adults (Post et al., 1993). However, the role of carbamazepine in treating adolescents needs to be studied better (Green, 1991).

ANXIETY DISORDERS

Clinical experience suggests that panic disorder and other anxiety disorders are very common in suicidal adolescents and adults. Mattison (1988) reported on several studies that demonstrate high levels of anxiety in suicidal adolescents and a high prevalence of suicidal thoughts in anxious adolescent patients. In a study of female adolescent suicide attempters, generalized anxiety disorder, separation anxiety, and simple phobia were common (14–28 percent), although not significantly more so than in nonattempting disturbed and nondisturbed controls (Trautman et al., 1991). Like dysthymia, anxiety disorders may have a chronic course. As a result, teenagers or parents may find it difficult spontaneously or readily to describe specific anxiety symptoms. Self-report screening questionnaires also will be of limited diagnostic value, because of limited self-awareness. Therefore, a clinical diagnostic interview must inquire specifically about symptoms of panic disorder and obsessive compulsive disorder.

Panic Disorder

Case 6

Barney was a 17-year-old high school junior who presented for treatment of panic attacks. In fact, for the past year he had had daily episodes of abrupt onset of panic, tachycardia, shortness of breath, depersonalization, chest pressure, and fears of losing control. During one of those episodes, he made a superficial laceration on his wrist. Although not suffering from a major depression, he was having arguments with his girlfriend, and was now feeling hopeless and angry, with suicidal thoughts. Clonazepam 0.5 mg tid was effective in stopping the panic attacks and in allowing psychotherapeutic consideration of his concerns about social and family relationships.

Although panic disorder is not often diagnosed in children and adolescents, it actually may be common (Moreau & Weissman, 1992). In adults, panic disorder frequently is associated with suicidal thoughts and attempts (Lepine, Chignon, & Teherani, 1993; Weissman, Klerman, Markowitz, & Ouellette, 1989). In a large epidemiologic sample of randomly selected adults, Weissman and associates (1989) found that 20 percent of subjects with panic disorder and 12 percent of those with panic attacks had made suicide attempts, as compared with only 6 percent for other psychiatric disorders. Panic symptoms frequently are misdiagnosed as severe anxiety, atypical asthma, or a myriad of other medical symptoms. Panic disorder often will be exacerbated by real or symbolic separations, such as parental divorce or conflict (Hendin, 1991). Overwhelming anticipatory anxiety and family turmoil can obscure the symptomatic role of panic attacks and their contribution to impulsive thoughts and behaviors. Self-medication with alcohol or drugs may reduce anxiety and obscure panic symptoms, and thereby further complicate accurate diagnosis.

Many medications are used for panic disorder. Tricyclic antidepressants are the best known (Klerman, 1992) but should be used cautiously, as noted earlier. Fluoxetine may decrease the frequency and severity of panic but may not eliminate attacks. While only two benzodiazepines are clearly effective for panic disorder, they start to work right away, rather than with the two- to four-week onset latency of antidepressant medications. Alprazolam (Klerman, 1992) is the only drug approved by the Food and Drug Administration (FDA) for treating panic disorder, but it is addicting, short acting, and difficult to taper. Rapid, short-term management of panic attacks often can be achieved more safely with clonazepam, another benzodiazepine. The longer half-life of clonazepam and absence of an induced euphoria help to reduce the likelihood of medication abuse and withdrawal. A tricyclic antidepressant may be substituted later for clonazepam once a therapeutic alliance has been formed and the crisis situation has come under control.

Anticipatory anxiety shows rapid improvement following cessation of panic attacks. Occasionally, in the absence of effective psychotherapy and patient education, there can be a paradoxical response to relief of panic attacks. The longer that some patients unwittingly experience a panic-free state, the more anticipatory anxiety there can be. This problem can be reduced by careful patient education about the relationship between panic attacks and anticipatory anxiety. Once panic attacks are treated successfully, psychodynamic issues of separation anxiety and rage frequently emerge in the therapy and may be addressed successfully. Often these issues in the adolescent relate to separation from parents, emerging independence, and the formation of an adult identity.

Obsessive Compulsive Disorder

Case 7

Carl was a 16-year-old tenth grader referred for treatment of depression and compulsions, particularly a need to "keep things symmetrical." He recalled that as early as age five he felt a need to touch things and later worried about stepping on cracks. His symptoms waxed and waned during early childhood. In seventh grade, he entered therapy because of sadness, sullenness, social withdrawal, and declining school grades. By ninth grade he was very preoccupied with "mental balance." While riding in a car he felt compelled to count telephone poles and driveways passing on each side. He was unable to play soccer because he couldn't keep track of his body's turns to the left and right sides. In class, these thoughts interfered with his concentration, and his grades again declined. Soon after, following disagreements with teachers and his girlfriend, he secretly took two aspirin overdoses. Carl found little enjoyment the next summer and complained of middle insomnia and fatigue. He felt guilty about spending too much time at his computer and too little at homework. There was no change, though, in his appetite or sexual interest.

Fluoxetine 20 mg daily was started, and raised to 40 mg after two weeks. After six weeks, Carl was sleeping better, was less tired, more cheerful, and less preoccupied with mental balance. He was still counting telephone poles. School grades improved substantially compared to the previous year. In the following months he complained that fluoxetine made him feel tired, but that if he took it at bedtime, he couldn't sleep. He began to take it irregularly, and while his mood remained good, the obsessions and compulsions increased. Although he was reluctant to change medications, the addition of trazodone 25 mg at bedtime improved his sleep.

Obsessive compulsive disorder (OCD) often is associated with profound isolation and embarrassment. Consequently, teenagers are typically ashamed of and reluctant to disclose obsessive compulsive symptoms. Symptoms of this disorder are manifest similarly in adults and adolescents: persistent and repetitive thoughts that intrude the thought process, and repetitive, stereotyped rituals. Rapoport and associates (1981) reported suicidal ideation in six of nine children with OCD. Individuals with obsessional thoughts and compulsions tend to be controlled and rigid. Impulsive responses to overwhelming obsessions and compulsions may occur.

Effective pharmacologic treatment for obsessive compulsive disorder is a relatively recent development and appears to be related to potentiation of the serotonin system. Fluoxetine (a selective serotonin reuptake inhibitor) and clomipramine (a tricyclic antidepressant) are both FDA approved for OCD and appear to be about equally effective (Green, 1991; Rasmussen, Eisen, & Pato, 1993). Fluoxetine is less likely than clomipramine to cause such common side effects as sedation and dry mouth and such rare events as seizure induction. Additional cautions for clomipramine are similar to the other tricyclics discussed earlier. Newer selective serotonin reuptake inhibitors, such as fluvoxamine, may prove effective also. Importantly, OCD medication response is often incomplete. Optimal treatment requires concurrent psychotherapy, behavior therapy, or both.

SCHIZOPHRENIA AND OTHER PSYCHOSES

Psychosis is a major risk factor for suicidal behavior. Therefore, a central clinical task in evaluating suicidal adolescents is to identify psychotic thinking, particularly command auditory hallucinations. Such symptoms usually will require inpatient management. Symptoms that emerge in the prodromal period of schizophrenia often are diagnosed (perhaps accurately) as indicative of depression, anxiety disorders, obsessive compulsive disorder, organic or toxic states, substance abuse, or borderline personality disorder. In particular, adolescents may show a gradual deterioration of personality, social withdrawal, declining performance, reduced motivation, and impaired self-esteem resembling depression. Sometimes only prolonged observation can resolve the diagnostic uncertainties. First-rank symptoms described by Schneider

(1959) are useful in establishing a diagnosis of schizophrenia in the adolescent age group. These symptoms include auditory hallucinations, delusions, and the belief that thoughts or feelings are controlled by outside forces.

Case 8

Harriet was a 15-year-old high school sophomore who was found wandering in traffic, and acknowledged fantasies of being hit by a car. For about a year she had been increasingly withdrawn. She had become preoccupied with the notion that demons infested her hair. On interview, she acknowledged that she sometimes heard a voice that commented on her behavior. She also described panic attacks, which seemed to make the voice and preoccupations worse. On haloperidol 2 mg bid and clonazepam 0.5 mg bid, she showed a prompt resolution of her symptoms and relief of her suicidal thoughts.

As in adults, neuroleptics are the first choice for pharmacologic treatment of adolescent schizophrenia. Low-potency neuroleptics, such as chlorpromazine and thioridazine, are associated with sedation and autonomic side effects, including orthostatic hypotension and tachycardia. High-potency neuroleptics such as haloperidol and fluphenazine are associated with extrapyramidal side effects, including parkinsonism, dystonias, and akathisia. Neuroleptic malignant syndrome is a life-threatening condition that may occur in the context of neuroleptic administration, and requires immediate medical intervention. A careful determination of the clinical grounds for neuroleptic administration in the adolescent is important because of the risk of tardive dyskinesia, a potentially irreversible side effect.

Adjunctive lithium can substantially enhance clinical response when psychosis occurs in the context of manic illness. Antidepressants and neuroleptics together can treat major depressive illness with psychotic symptoms successfully. Kahn, Puertollano, Schane, and Klein (1988) reported on seven patients with schizophrenia and panic attacks whose positive and negative schizophrenic symptoms all improved markedly when alprazolam was added to their antipsychotic medication regimen.

TREATMENT AND COMPLIANCE

Adolescents with medication-responsive syndromes require careful diagnosis, treatment, and follow-up management. Effective relief of symptoms often will bring an acute suicidal crisis under control and may open the way for effective individual and family therapy. Medication management, however, is not a substitute for psychotherapy. Any suicidal adolescent is struggling with major emotional issues, typically relating to maturation, loss, separation, or complex family dynamics. In the absence of a therapeutic alliance and appropriate psychotherapy with a suicidal adolescent, there is a greater likelihood of medication noncompliance, potentially fatal overdose of prescribed medications, continued substance abuse, and inadequate resolution of pressing emotional concerns.

Compliance with treatment is one of the overriding issues in therapy. Litt, Cuskey, and Rudd (1983) found that adolescent compliance with initial referral from an emergency room is as low as 33 percent. Further, even those teenagers who do present for outpatient treatment are unlikely to continue. Poor compliance with follow-up is a particular concern for medication management in the suicidal adolescent, where appropriate drug monitoring and ongoing assessment of patient safety are paramount.

Trautman, Stewart, and Morishima (1993) reviewed the problem of adolescent compliance with follow-up treatment. They suggested that noncompliance can stem from a teenager's conscious awareness that suicidal ideation or gestures are intended as a deliberate manipulation and that he or she does not actually want professional help. On a diagnostic level, a noncompliant adolescent may harbor depressive nihilism, phobic avoidance, or psychotic fears. Individuals with antisocial or paranoid personality traits may be particularly difficult to engage in a therapeutic alliance. Finally, noncompliance often is an attempt to prevent interference with drug or alcohol abuse.

Complex family dynamics also may interfere with a suicidal adolescent's compliance with treatment. Rotheram-Borus and Trautman (1988) reported that 70 percent of adolescent girls attempting suicide did so following an argument with their parents. Parents may overtly or covertly discourage treatment because they themselves may have similar and untreated psychiatric problems and may resent a diagnostic label and treatment for the child. Furthermore, the parents may see chronic depressive or anxiety syndromes as a condition that must be endured, rather than treated. Parental self-medication with drugs or alcohol, stoic forbearance of psychiatric symptoms, and even suicidal behavior also can set an example that the teenager follows, rather than seeking out or accepting treatment. Last, many parents grapple with fears and feelings of guilt that they are responsible for causing their teenager's problems, either emotionally or through genetic inheritance.

Parents of suicidal teenagers may be particularly unaware of their child's suicidal thoughts or dysphoric symptoms (Walker, Moreau, & Weissman, 1990; Zimmerman & Asnis, 1991). This unawareness can result from parental denial, emotional detachment, poor parent-child communication, depression, projected hopelessness, or even unconscious hostility toward the child. Careful parental education about concrete details of symptoms, diagnosis, treatment, and prognosis is essential. Engagement of the parents, from the first session, is as essential as engagement of the adolescent if treatment is to succeed. Equally careful attention needs to be given to the dynamics of family interactions.

Suicidal thoughts and actions often serve such defensive purposes as seeking help or attention, angry retaliation through communication of suffering, or efforts at stabilizing parental marital discord. Consequently, the child may feel an emotional need to hold on to otherwise painful psychiatric symptoms. In particular, a need to defy seemingly uncaring or hostile authorities is a major barrier to medication compliance. This is especially true if the psychiatrist is seen exclusively as an agent of the parents. Further, even with effective medication treatment of a psychiatric disorder, the adolescent may continue to experience suicidal ideation.

Finally, even fully cooperative parents often will have strong feelings about medication treatment for their child. Parents will be concerned about possible side effects, overdose, or risk that medication use would lead to drug or alcohol abuse. Some parents may view medications as a "crutch" or as a way of avoiding "real" problems.

SUMMARY

There is much research yet to be done in medication management of the suicidal adolescent; psychopharmacologic intervention in adolescent suicide is still not well understood. Careful attention to the psychopharmacologic component of treatment includes several tasks. Accurate diagnosis requires a careful and specific clinical interview. Ascertainment of diagnosis allows selection of medication specific to diagnosis. Treatment compliance is encouraged through the therapeutic alliance and through attention to individual and family psychodynamics. Finally, treatment response and side effects are observed carefully, with attention as well to the emotional conflicts triggered by medication response. All of these tasks are complicated by the fact that suicidal adolescents may be defiant of authority, enmeshed in complex family dynamics, continuing substance abuse, and struggling with many and complex developmental concerns. Nevertheless, it is clear that psychopharmacological intervention can help, especially in conjunction with psychotherapy.

REFERENCES

American Psychiatric Association. (1994). *Diagnostic and statistical manual of mental disorders* (4th ed.) (DSM-IV). Washington, DC: American Psychiatric Association.

Asnis, G. M., McGinn, L. K., & Sanderson, W. C. (in press). Atypical depression: Clinical aspects and noradrenergic function. *American Journal of Psychiatry*.

Baldessarini, R. (1990). Drugs and the treatment of psychiatric disorders. In A. Gilman, T. Rall, A. Nies, & P. Taylor (Eds.), *The pharmacological basis of therapeutics* (8th ed., pp. 383–435). New York: Pergamon Press.

Boulos, C., Kutcher, S., Gardner, D., & Young, E. (1992). An open naturalistic trial of fluoxetine in adolescents and young adults with treatment-resistant major depression. *Journal of Child and Adolescent Psychopharmacology, 2*(2), 103–111.

Brent, D. A., Kalas, R., Edelbrock, C., Costello, A. J., Dulcan, M. K., & Conover, N. (1986). Psychopathology and its relationship to suicidal ideation in childhood and adolescence. *Journal of the American Academy of Child and Adolescent Psychiatry, 25*(5), 666–673.

Brent, D. A., Perper, J. A., Goldstein, C. E., Kolko, D. J., Allan, M. J., Allman, C. J., & Zelenak, J. P. (1988). Risk factors for adolescent suicide: A comparison of adolescent suicide victims with suicidal inpatients. *Archives of General Psychiatry, 45*, 581–588.

Brent, D. A., Perper, J. A., Moritz, G., Allman, C., Friend, A., Roth, C., Schweers, J., Balach, L., & Baugher, M. (1993). Psychiatric risk factors for adolescent suicide: A case-control study. *Journal of the American Academy of Child and Adolescent Psychiatry, 32*(3), 521–529.

Carlson, G., Davenport, Y., & Jamison, K. (1977). A comparison of outcome in adolescent and late-onset bipolar manic-depressive illness. *American Journal of Psychiatry, 134,* 919–922.

DeLong, G. R., & Aldershof, A. L. (1987). Long-term experience with lithium treatment in childhood: Correlation with clinical diagnosis. *Journal of the American Academy of Child and Adolescent Psychiatry, 26,* 389–394.

Green, W. H. (1991). Antidepressants. In M. G. Fisher (Ed.), *Child and adolescent clinical psychopharmacology.* Baltimore, MD: Williams and Wilkins.

Harrison, W. M., & Stewart, J. W. (1993). Pharmacotherapy of dysthymia. *Psychiatric Annals, 23,* 638–648.

Hendin, H. (1991). Psychodynamics of suicide, with particular reference to the young. *American Journal of Psychiatry, 148,* 1150–1158.

Hirsch, S. R., Walsh, C., & Draper, R. (1982). Parasuicide. *Journal of Affective Disorders, 4,* 299–311.

Kahn, J. P., Puertollano, M. A., Schane, M. D., & Klein, D. F. (1988). Adjunctive alprazolam for schizophrenia with panic anxiety: Clinical observation and pathogenetic implications. *American Journal of Psychiatry, 145,* 742–744.

Keller, M. B., Lavori, P. W., Beardslee, W. R., Wunder, J., & Ryan, N. (1991). Depression in children and adolescents: New data on "undertreatment" and a literature review on the efficacy of available treatments. *Journal of Affective Disorders, 21,* 163–171.

Klerman, G. (1992). Drug treatment of panic disorder: Comparative efficacy of alprazolam, imipramine, and placebo. *British Journal of Psychiatry, 160,* 191–202.

Kovacs, M., Feinberg, T. L., Crouse-Novak, M. A., Paulauskas, S. L., & Finkelstein, R. (1984). Depressive disorders in childhood I: A longitudinal prospective study of characteristics and recovery. *Archives of General Psychiatry, 41,* 229–237.

Leenaars, A. A., & Wenckstern, S. (1991). *Suicide prevention in schools.* New York: Hemisphere Publishing Corporation.

Lepine, J. P., Chignon, J. M., & Teherani, M. (1993). Suicide attempts in patients with panic disorder. *Archives of General Psychiatry, 50,* 144–149.

Litt, I., Cuskey, W., & Rudd, S. (1983). Emergency room evaluation of the adolescent who attempts suicide: Compliance with follow-up. *Journal of Adolescent Health Care, 4,* 106–108.

Martunnen, M. J., Aro, H. M., Henriksson, M. M., & Lonnqvist, J. K. (1991). Mental disorders in adolescent suicide: DSM-III-R axes I and

II diagnoses in suicides among 13- to 19-year olds in Finland. *Archives of General Psychiatry, 48,* 834–839.

Mattison, R. (1988). Suicide and other consequences of childhood and adolescent anxiety disorders. *Journal of Clinical Psychiatry, 49*(10, Suppl.), 9–11.

McBride, P. A., Trautman, P. D., & Glick, I. Unpublished raw data.

Moreau, D., & Weissman, M. M. (1992). Panic disorder in children and adolescents: A review. *American Journal of Psychiatry, 149,* 1306–1314.

Myers, K., McCauley, E., Calderon, R., Mitchell, J., Burke, P., & Schloredt, K. (1991). Risks for suicidality in major depressive disorder. *Journal of the American Academy of Child and Adolescent Psychiatry, 30*(1), 86–94.

Olsen, T. (1961). Follow-up study of manic-depressive patients whose first attack occurred before the age of 19 years. *Acta Psychiatrica Scandinavia, 162* (Suppl.), 45–51.

Pande, A. C., Haskett, R. F., & Graden, J. F. (1992, June). *Fluoxetine treatment of atypical depression.* Paper presented at the 145th Annual Meeting of the American Psychiatric Association. Washington, DC.

Pfeffer, C. R., Klerman, G. L., Hurt, S. W., Lesser, M., Peskin, J. R., & Siefker, C.A. (1991). Suicidal children grow up: Demographic and clinical risk factors for adolescent suicide attempts. *Journal of the American Academy of Child and Adolescent Psychiatry, 30*(4), 609–616.

Pfeffer, C. R., Peskin, J. R., & Siefker, C. A. (1992). Suicidal children grow up: Psychiatric treatment during follow-up period. *Journal of the American Academy of Child and Adolescent Psychiatry, 31*(4), 679–685.

Physicians' Desk Reference (48th ed.) (1994). Oradell, NJ: Medical Economics Co.

Post, R. M., Keller, T. A., Pazzaglia, P. J., George, M. S., Marangell, L., & Denicoff, K. (1993). New developments in the use of anticonvulsants as mood stabilizers. *Neuropsychobiology, 27*(3), 132–137.

Preskorn, S. H., Weller, E. B., & Weller, R. A. (1982). Depression in children: Relationship between plasma imipramine levels and response. *Journal of Clinical Psychiatry, 43,* 450–453.

Puig-Antich, J., Perel, J. M., Lupatkin, W., Chambers, W. J., Shea, C., Tabrizi, M. D., & Stiller, B. (1979). Plasma levels of imipramine (IMI) and desmethylimipramine (DMI) and clinical response in prepubertal major depressive disorder: A preliminary report. *Journal of the American Academy of Child and Adolescent Psychiatry, 18,* 616–627.

Puig-Antich, J., Perel, J. M., Lupatkin, W., Chambers, W. J., Tabrizi, M. A., King, J., Goetz, R., Davies, M., & Stiller, R. L. (1987). Imipramine in prepubertal major depressive disorders. *Archives of General Psychiatry, 44,* 81–89.

Quitkin, F. M., McGrath, P., Stewart, J., Harrison, W., Wager, S., Nunes, E., Rabkin, J., Tricamo, E., Markowitz, J., & Klein, D. (1989). Phenelzine and imipramine in mood reactive depressives: Further delineation of the syndrome of atypical depression. *Archives of General Psychiatry, 46*(9), 787–793.

Rapoport, J., Elkins, R., Langer, D., Sceery, W., Buchsbaum, M. S., Gillin, J. C., Murphy, D. L., Zahn, T. P., Lake, R., Ludlow, C., & Mendelson, W. (1988). Childhood obsessive compulsive disorder. *American Journal of Psychiatry, 138,* 1545–1554.

Rasmussen, S. A., Eisen, J. L., & Pato, M. T. (1993). Current issues in the pharmacologic management of obsessive compulsive disorder. *Journal of Clinical Psychiatry, 54*(6, Suppl.), 4–9.

Riddle, M. A., Nelson, J. C., Kleinman, C. S., Rasmusson, A., Leckman, J. F., King, R. A., & Cohen, D. J. (1991). Sudden death in children receiving norpramin: A review of three reported cases and commentary. *Journal of the American Academy of Child and Adolescent Psychiatry, 30*(1), 104–107.

Rotheram-Borus, M. J., & Trautman, P. (1988). Hopelessness, depression, and suicidal intent among adolescent suicide attempters. *Journal of the American Academy of Child and Adolescent Psychiatry, 27,* 700–704.

Rutter, M., & Hersov, L. (Eds.) (1985). *Child and adolescent psychiatry: Modern approaches.* Boston, MA: Blackwell Scientific Publications.

Ryan, N. D., Puig-Antich, J., Cooper, T. B., Rabinovich, H., Ambrosini, P., Davies, M., King, J., Torres, D., & Fried, J. (1986). Imipramine in adolescent major depression: Plasma level and clinical response. *Acta Psychiatrica Scandanavia, 73,* 275–288.

Schneider, K. (1959). *Clinical psychopathology.* New York: Grune & Stratton.

Shaffer, D., Garland, A., Gould, M., Fisher, P., & Trautman, P. (1988). Preventing teenage suicide: A critical review. *Journal of the American Academy of Child and Adolescent Psychiatry, 27*(6), 675–687.

Shaffi, M., Carrigan, S., Whittinghill, J. R., & Derrick, A. (1985). Psychological autopsy of completed suicide in children and adolescents. *American Journal of Psychiatry, 142,* 1061–1064.

Strober, M., Freeman, R., & Rigali, J. (1990). The pharmacotherapy of depressive illness in adolescence I: An open label trial of imipramine. *Psychopharmacology Bulletin, 26,* 80–84.

Strober, M., Morrell, W., Burroughs, J., Lampert, C., Danforth, H., & Freeman, R. (1988). A family study of bipolar I disorder in adolescence: Early onset of symptoms linked to increased familial loading and lithium resistance. *Journal of Affective Disorders, 15*(3), 255–268.

Strober, M., Morrell, W., Lampert, C., & Burroughs, J. (1990). Relapse following discontinuation of lithium maintenance therapy in adolescents with bipolar I illness: A naturalistic study. *American Journal of Psychiatry, 147,* 457–461.

Trautman, P. D., Rotheram-Borus, M. J., Dopkins, S., & Lewin, N. (1991). Psychiatric diagnoses in minority female adolescent suicide attempters. *Journal of the American Academy of Child and Adolescent Psychiatry, 30*(4), 617–622.

Trautman, P., & Shaffer, D. (1984). Treatment of child and adolescent suicide attempters. In H. Sudak, A. Ford, & N. Rushforth (Eds.). *Suicide in the young* (pp. 307–323). Boston: John Wright PSG.

Trautman, P. D., Stewart, N., & Morishima, A. (1993). Are adolescent suicide attempters noncompliant with outpatient care? *Journal of the American Academy of Child and Adolescent Psychiatry, 32,* 89–94.

Walker, M., Moreau, D., & Weissman, M. M. (1990). Parents' awareness of children's suicide attempts. *American Journal of Psychiatry, 147,* 1364–1366.

Weissman, M. M., Klerman, G. L., Markowitz, J. S., & Ouellette, R. (1989). Suicidal ideation and suicide attempts in panic disorder and attacks. *New England Journal of Medicine, 321,* 1209–1214.

Welner, A., Welner, Z., & Fishman, R. (1979). Psychiatric adolescent inpatients: Eight- to ten-year follow-up. *Archives of General Psychiatry, 36,* 698–700.

Zimmerman, J. K., & Asnis, G. M. (1991). Parents' knowledge of children's suicide attempts: Awareness or denial? *American Journal of Psychiatry, 148*(8), 1091–1092.

13

Long-Term Follow-Up with Suicidal Adolescents
A Clinical Perspective

MARTHA E. WOODARD AND
JAMES K. ZIMMERMAN

Past research indicates that a suicide attempt in adolescence is one of the most consistent risk factors for repeated attempts and completed suicide (Davidson & Linnoila, 1989; Holinger, 1989; Pfeffer, 1989; Pfeffer et al., 1991; Pfeffer et al., 1993; Spirito, 1990; Spirito, Brown, Overholser, & Fritz, 1989). However, some research suggests that many outreach efforts do not succeed in preventing adolescent suicide or reducing suicidal behavior because they are directed at teenagers in general instead of being focally targeted at adolescents at risk for suicide (Shaffer et al., 1991; Shaffer et al., 1990; Vieland, Whittle, Garland, Hicks, & Shaffer, 1991). Further, other studies have shown that adolescent suicide attempters often are lost to psychiatric follow-up after referral for further treatment and are unlikely to attend and complete indicated treatment (Hengeveld, van Egmond, Bouwmans, & van Rooyen, 1991; Litt, Cuskey, & Rudd, 1983; Nardini-Maillard & Ladame, 1980; Rotheram, 1990; Spirito et al., 1989; Spirito et al., 1992; Trautman & Rotheram, 1986; Trautman & Stewart, 1989). Some studies do suggest, however, that frequency and timeliness of contact may influence compliance (e.g., Clarke, 1988; Frankel & Hovell, 1978).

Unfortunately, due to the difficulties involved in contacting and engaging this population, few studies have followed adolescents systematically after a suicide attempt (Pfeffer et al., 1991; Pfeffer, Peskin, & Siefker, 1992; Spirito et al., 1992). This lack of both research studies and clinical follow-up programs is of particular concern considering the risk among adolescents of recidivistic suicidal behavior and the potential for completed suicides if clinical interventions are not made in a timely manner. Clearly, if adolescents are unlikely to comply with treatment or respond to follow-up protocols, effective intervention becomes more difficult.

In developing and implementing a follow-up procedure with suicidal adolescents, there are practical problems encountered in addition to those created by the psychosocial issues these individuals manifest. These include change of address, lack of telephone or its disconnection, frequency of moves, and so on (Nardini-Maillard & Ladame, 1980; Spirito, 1990). Reich and Earls (1990) state that a common frustration in longitudinal procedures is that the recipients of contact become more widely dispersed over time and subsequently more difficult, time-consuming, and expensive to track.

Thus, without finding a way to contact and engage suicidal adolescents who are nonresponders to follow-up and noncompliers with treatment, the validity and usefulness of prospective studies are questionable and the ability to develop and implement effective prevention and treatment for this population is minimal at best.

TELEPHONE AS METHOD OF FOLLOW-UP

Telephone surveys have been found to be a cost-effective alternative to personal interviewing; however, only a few studies to date have examined the effectiveness of the telephone as both a clinical and research tool for follow-up. Tausig and Freeman (1988) found, in a group of women who were patients in an in vitro fertilization and embryo transfer program, that approximately 70 percent responded to follow-up after 15 months, as opposed to 31 percent and 50 percent response rates in face-to-face follow-up studies (Hengeveld et al., 1991). Additionally, all but two of the 156 participants consented to be contacted for continued follow-up at a future date. Patients did not view the telephone interviews as intrusive, but rather as a "welcome opportunity" to talk about their experiences (Tausig & Freeman, 1988, p. 424). Besides the cost-effectiveness and convenience for the participant, it was hypothesized that another advantage of telephone contact is that visual anonymity may reduce the self-consciousness that often characterizes personal interviews.

In a study comparing live and telephone interviews, Paulsen, Crowe, Noyes, and Pfohl (1988) investigated families of patients with panic disorders. They found a high level of agreement between diagnoses made in person and by telephone and concluded that lifetime diagnoses of panic disorder, major depression, and alcohol abuse in adults reliably could be made in a family study using the telephone interview.

In another study employing a structured psychiatric interview, Reich and Earls (1990) compared groups of adolescents interviewed by telephone and in person. There were no significant differences in the reporting of diagnoses or personal information between the two groups; however, the telephone group as a whole reported fewer symptoms than did the group interviewed in person. Despite this difference, these researchers concluded that telephone interviews with adolescents "may be a useful methodological strategy in studies where face-to-face interviews . . . are difficult if not impossible to obtain" (Reich & Earls, 1990, p. 214).

In another recent study using the telephone interview as a tool for follow-up, Spirito and associates (1992) contacted adolescents and their parents by telephone one and three months following a suicide attempt. The goal of this prospective short-term study was to assess various areas of psychosocial dysfunction, repeat suicide attempts, and treatment compliance in adolescent suicide attempters. The response rate was 81 percent at one month and 80 percent at the three month interview. Despite these high response rates, skepticism was expressed about the advantages of telephone interviews over face-to-face follow-up. Unlike Tausig and Freeman (1988), Spirito and coworkers (1992) were concerned that telephone interviews may limit the individual's willingness to speak openly about personal information.

Although past research on telephone follow-up with adolescents is sparse, findings such as those just presented suggest that this method may be an effective alternative to interviews in person in several ways:

1. Since suicidal adolescents often do not access mental health services, telephone follow-up may be a way of maintaining contact with those who would not otherwise receive any services. This may reduce recidivism if a working alliance can be established by telephone such that the adolescent is more likely to rely on mental health services in times of crisis.

2. Response rates to telephone contact may be higher than those to face-to-face interviews that require a clinic appointment.

3. Adolescents may feel more comfortable with telephone contact in part because this mode of communication is so commonly used by them (Reich & Earls, 1990).

4. Telephone contact is a cost- and labor-effective use of a clinician's time.

The focus of this chapter is to consider the use of telephone follow-up as a clinical intervention. Consequently, the next section describes briefly the implementation of a telephone follow-up procedure (the PFPEP) in an inner-city outpatient clinic offering time-limited treatment (approximately three months' duration) for depressed and suicidal adolescents. Following that, suggestions for the use of telephone follow-up as a form of clinical outreach are presented.

IMPLEMENTATION OF THE PFPEP

The Patient Follow-up and Program Evaluation Protocol (PFPEP) was implemented as a consequence of concerns over the long-term risk of recidivism in suicidal adolescents and because of the recognition that many of these individuals were not compliant with scheduled appointments for outpatient mental health treatment. The PFPEP was intended both to prevent recidivism by developing ongoing relationships with at-risk individuals (as per recommendations made by Shaffer et al., 1990) and to evaluate the effects of treatment in the clinic. Although less structured telephone follow-up had taken place previously, the establishment of the PFPEP made patient follow-up an integral part of treatment in an effort to maintain contact with the high-risk population with which the clinic staff had contact.

The initial intent of the PFPEP was to elucidate two issues: to investigate the impact of attendance in the clinic on subsequent suicidal behavior, depressive symptoms, and psychosocial and family functioning; and to determine if more frequent follow-up contact decreases recidivism and increases accessibility of adolescents to later structured interviews. All adolescents referred to the clinic were followed by telephone after their contact with the program, regardless of whether they were actually treated in the program. They were contacted for a structured interview by telephone at six months and at one year after last clinic contact. (For a more complete description of methodology, refer to Zimmerman and Woodard, 1993.) The interview included ratings of depression and suicidal symptomatology (employing subscales from the K-SADS [Schedule for Affective Disorders and Schizophrenia—Children's Version; Chambers et al., 1985]) and psychosocial functioning (including family, peer group, and academic functioning as well as involvement in conduct disordered behavior and substance abuse). To examine the influence of frequency of contact (as per the suggestions of Clarke, 1988; Frankel & Hovell, 1978), half of the adolescents participating in the PFPEP were contacted on a monthly basis for the first year in addition to the more comprehensive six-month and one-year interviews. This monthly contact was brief, including ratings on depression and suicidal ideation and questions regarding upcoming changes of address or telephone.

RESULTS OF IMPLEMENTATION OF PFPEP

Although the focus of this chapter is on the clinical use of telephone follow-up, several findings reported elsewhere (Zimmerman & Woodard, 1993) are worthy of mention here. First of all, the implementation of the PFPEP significantly increased compliance with telephone follow-up over the previous year. This is most likely due to the fact that follow-up was more formalized and consistently implemented on an ongoing basis under the PFPEP. Further, patients and their parents were told in advance to expect that they would be contacted by telephone by clinic staff, and this may have helped increase compliance as well.

Second, attendance in the clinic was related to decreased depression and suicidality upon six-month follow-up as well as with increased satisfaction with certain interpersonal relationships. Although these findings cannot be attributed definitively to positive effects of treatment in the clinic without further research, there were demonstrable differences over a six-month period between adolescents who received treatment and those who did not, despite the fact that the groups did not differ demographically or with regard to suicidal ideation and attempts before initial contact with the clinic. Those who attended appointments tended to be more likely to participate in the PFPEP as well.

Third, frequency of contact during the first six months of the PFPEP did not affect compliance with follow-up. This suggests that less frequent contact, which would allow for more efficient use of staff time, could be employed in future telephone follow-up efforts with suicidal adolescents. However, it should be noted that frequent contact was instrumental in helping some adolescents access psychotherapeutic services, in many cases for the first time. Utilizing the PFPEP allowed a relationship to be maintained with adolescents who may not have received any mental health intervention otherwise; this suggests that such an approach can target and intervene with adolescents who are difficult to access in other ways (Shaffer et al., 1990; Shaffer et al., 1991; Vieland et al., 1991).

THE NEED FOR INTERVENTION

In addition to the findings just presented, 28 percent of adolescents contacted were interested in further psychotherapy for themselves, and 24 percent of parents were interested in treatment for their children. In 15 cases, a crisis was occurring or had recently occurred when the follow-up telephone call was made. Five of these adolescents in crisis were referred to a hospital emergency room, and five were readmitted to the clinic. The remaining five were referred to their catchment area clinic for further treatment.

It is also significant to note that a substantial number of adolescents who were referred to the clinic but who did not receive treatment there were aided by telephone contact. Eleven of these adolescents (34 percent) were interested in treatment upon contact, as were nine of their parents. Since these adolescents are among those who otherwise would have "fallen through the cracks" in the mental health system, these findings suggest that the outreach component of the PFPEP and similar follow-up efforts has the potential for significant impact in reducing the incidence of suicidal behavior in adolescents.

RESTRUCTURING OF THE PFPEP

The need for intervention, which was expressed by a substantial number of adolescents and parents who participated in the PFPEP, led to a revision of the purposes of the follow-up. It became clear within a month after implementation that the original intents of the project—to evaluate the effects of clinic treatment and determine if frequency of contact had an impact on adolescent compliance with follow-up—needed to be expanded because many of the adolescents and their family members contacted were either in crisis and/or requested further services. The original role of the caller as "interviewer" and "researcher" quickly diversified to include "crisis worker," "case manager," "therapist," and "consultant." These roles occurred intermittently, sometimes consecutively, and frequently simultaneously.

The following sections describe first the types of outreach services requested by parents and then those requested by adolescents. The hope is that these descriptions and clinical vignettes will stimulate innovative research and clinical interventions in the areas of follow-up and outreach services with suicidal adolescents.

CONTACT WITH PARENTS

Although families received a letter about the PFPEP before the first telephone call, direct contact was attempted with all parents in order to inform parents of the nature of the project, to gain their support for the PFPEP, to assuage any concerns they might have, and to defer to their parental authority. In addition to discussing the intent of the calls and issues of confidentiality, the interviewer always informed parents that if they needed any assistance concerning their adolescents, they could call the interviewer directly. Overall, parents were both receptive and appreciative of the telephone contact. Furthermore, few adolescents complained about parental contact; in fact, many adolescents expressed conflict concerning their family relationships and were happy and occasionally eager to have the interviewer talk to their parents. Because family conflict has been found to be one of the risk factors in adolescent suicide attempts (see Pfeffer, 1989, and Spirito et al., 1989, for reviews of the literature), this eagerness was not surprising. Additionally, because guidelines about confidentiality were explained during the initial call to both parents and adolescents, confusion and misunderstanding regarding this issue generally were avoided.

The types of parental contact that caused the interviewer to move away from a research stance and toward case management or crisis intervention were the following: parents seeking treatment for their child and parents needing crisis intervention. The approach taken to these requests is described next.

Requests for Treatment

Approximately 24 percent of parents contacted inquired about treatment for their adolescents. In a group of 18 parents for whom data are available, 11 (61 percent) of them followed through with treatment referrals made by the PFPEP interviewer—that is, they actually made and kept an appointment for therapy.

Besides inquiring about referral information, many parents wanted immediate support and advice over the telephone. These parents often described feeling helpless, hopeless, overwhelmed, and alone as they struggled with how best to help their adolescent. As a result, brief and direct interventions were introduced to these parents over the telephone. These interventions, cognitive-behavioral in style, fell into three overall categories: problem-solving techniques; reframing and cognitive restructuring; and psychoeducation. The following sections provide brief examples of these interventions.

Problem-Solving Techniques

To enhance problem-solving abilities, the interviewer (M.W.) taught the parent how to "brainstorm," list, and explore a number of available options and to consider positive and negative consequences of each one. The intent of this intervention was to empower parents and help them make their own informed decisions.

Reframing and Restructuring

Parents often expressed guilt about their adolescent's situation, describing themselves as "bad parents" and "failures." In response, the interviewer pointed out the difference between state and trait; that is, that they might have acted in inappropriate ways, but that did not mean that they were "bad parents."

Psychoeducation

Additionally, the interviewer educated the parent about adolescent development and some issues that occur both individually for the adolescent and interpersonally between adolescents and their parents (e.g., separation-individuation, identity development, physical changes).

Not only did these interventions give parents new tools to cope more effectively with difficult situations and help put their current struggle with their adolescent in perspective, but the telephone call also helped them feel more supported and less isolated. Implicitly, we assumed that if parents felt more empowered and less "bad," they would be more effective in helping their child. The following cases illustrate the supportive role of the interviewer and the impact this had on the parent.

Case Example: José—Trouble in School

A 15-year-old Puerto Rican male, José, was referred to the clinic for depression and acting-out behaviors such as lying, stealing, and truancy. Because his behavior was chronic, and the clinic program was time-limited, he was referred directly for long-term treatment. He was randomly assigned to the monthly contact group; initial contact was made with his mother during the first month. She had not followed through on the initial referral for long-term treatment because her son's school problems had decreased. However, by the third monthly call, José's behavior had deteriorated such that he was cutting and failing most of his classes again and would most likely be left back. The interviewer suggested to the mother that she think about placing her son on the waiting list at a local mental health clinic and gave her the necessary information to make the call.

During the next monthly call, the mother stated that she was ambivalent about following through with the referral because she was worried both about her son's response and that she might not be doing the "right thing." The interviewer helped her assess the pros and cons of therapy for her son and what it meant for her to instigate it. On the fifth monthly call, the mother stated that she had scheduled an appointment for therapy for her son.

Case Example: Mary—A Grandmother's Strength

Mary, a 14-year-old black female, was not originally accepted into the clinic due to a chronic history of school truancy, delinquency, and running away; recommendations were made for either long-term outpatient treatment or a residential setting. The first follow-up interview with Mary was conducted at six months after referral. At that time, Mary's grandmother, her legal guardian, answered the telephone; she expressed appreciation for the interviewer's concern and stated that Mary was currently in treatment, but that the situation was still unstable.

Five months later, the grandmother initiated a call to the interviewer, stating that Mary had dropped out of treatment, had run away multiple times, had stopped attending school, and had been placed in two different group homes. The grandmother had been in contact with the court, judges, a lawyer, and various social workers connected with her case. At the time of the call, Mary had recently run away from another group home, and her grandmother wanted to get her into residential treatment. The grandmother had previously sought individual treatment for Mary, taken out a PINS (Person In Need of Supervision) petition, and had ongoing contact with the court and social services; these attempts were clearly to no avail, and had left the grandmother feeling frustrated and helpless in the face of a number of social services system problems such as overloaded caseworkers, overcrowded facilities, and unreturned telephone calls. The focus of the call was thus to help the grandmother find a more effective way to work within this system, not to add to this already large number of "helping professionals." The interviewer helped the grandmother create a new list of options she currently had available to her, such as first talking with the professional with whom she felt most comfortable in order to schedule a group meeting with all those involved in the case to come up with a plan of action, taking Mary to an emergency room for a psychiatric evaluation, taking out another PINS petition, and so on.

The grandmother was worried about whether placing her granddaughter in a residential treatment center was the "right" action to take, and felt Mary might "hate" her for it. The interviewer supported the grandmother's strength in working so hard to help Mary; the interviewer also emphasized that despite Mary's current anger, it was important that she had someone who loved and cared for her enough to "get her on the right track." The interviewer also helped the grandmother not to personalize Mary's anger.

At the time of the one-year call, one month later, the grandmother sounded more calm and focused. She had recently taken Mary to the emergency room for a psychiatric evaluation and was currently involved in the process of getting her hospitalized. She also was working with a number of professionals she trusted and felt were helping her. The interviewer supported these recent actions and her strength and commitment in continuing to help Mary. The grandmother stated that she appreciated the telephone calls because she felt like the interviewer was an ally and gave her the confidence she needed to keep going.

In the cases of both José and Mary, the interviewer played the role of the caregiver's ally. Both women expressed a sense of hopelessness and a feeling of failure as a caregiver. Similar approaches were used with both women. The interviewer listened and empathized with them, focused on their strengths, discussed their previous attempts at improving their situations, helped them to "brainstorm" about present options and analyze the potential consequences of these actions, and taught them how to counter their irrational beliefs. Most important, rather than getting directly involved, the interviewer encouraged these women to find a contact person within the system of professionals already involved in their case to whom they could turn for assistance. In this way, the interviewer remained on the periphery and was able to maintain the role of interviewer, rather than becoming yet another therapist or case manager in the lives of these women. As a result of the interviewer's interventions, both José's mother and Mary's grandmother felt more confident about their ability to manage their difficult situations and expressed more hope and clarity about their adolescent's future.

CONTACT WITH ADOLESCENTS

Consistent with the experience with parents, a large number of adolescents (28 percent) contacted by telephone expressed an interest in further psychotherapy. Again, 11 of 18 (61 percent) for whom data are available followed through with treatment recommendations.

In general, prior to giving any referral information to adolescents, the telephone interview was completed so that an initial assessment of the situation was made. In addition to being consistent with a research protocol, this allowed the interviewer to evaluate the adolescent's level of suicide risk and available support systems—information that was necessary for making an appropriate referral.

Along with referral information, a number of other issues were addressed. First, the interviewer asked the adolescent about parental involvement in treatment, both in order to facilitate intake into a mental health clinic and to increase the likelihood of treatment compliance (as per Spirito, 1990). Very few adolescents adamantly refused parental involvement; on the contrary, most wanted their parents involved, and many asked the interviewer to help them in this regard. Nevertheless, if the adolescent clearly did not want parental involvement and was not actively suicidal, the interviewer respected that choice.

Second, if the adolescent expressed openness to parental involvement, the interviewer asked permission to give referral information directly to the parent while assuring the adolescent that confidentiality would be respected (unless the adolescent was currently at risk of harm to self or others).

Third, the interviewer discussed with the adolescent what to expect once a call was made to schedule an appointment for treatment. The intent was to prepare the adolescent (and parents) to anticipate the frustrations and confusions attendant upon entering the community mental health system, so that compliance would be more likely to occur. Since many adolescents had assumed that they would call and immediately talk with someone about their problems, they were appreciative about being told what to expect in advance. In all cases, the interviewer reminded the adolescent to call back in the interim with any questions, concerns, or need for further assistance in the process of obtaining psychotherapeutic services.

Finally, the interviewer asked adolescents what might prevent them from successfully following through with the referral. In response, many adolescents expressed ambivalence about seeking help for themselves. Some of the most frequently mentioned reasons included a negative experience in previous treatment, fear of being crazy, fear that nothing will change, fear of parental involvement, lack of financial resources, and lack of trust in others. The interviewer discussed each concern with the adolescent, employing a direct cognitive challenge to the adolescent's irrational beliefs while supporting his or her problem-solving skills. For instance, with regard to the concern that prospective treatment would not be helpful because a previous experience was negative, the interviewer posed questions such as: Does one bad experience in treatment mean that all future experiences would be bad? What can the adolescent do to make this experience better? What precautions can be taken to ensure a better experience this time?

Another common misconception was that only "crazy" people need to see a therapist. The interviewer challenged this belief, conveying the message that seeking treatment is often a sign of strength. A further goal of this discussion was to educate the adolescent about the process of therapy. Topics that were frequently explored included: how talking helps, that there is no "miracle cure," that they might feel worse before they feel better, and expected length of treatment.

Finally, for adolescents who continued to express ambivalence, the interviewer helped create a list of reasons why treatment might and might not be helpful; this assisted them in clarifying potential treatment goals they themselves might support. The hope was that the more the adolescents were aware of potential pitfalls, the more likely they would become successfully engaged in treatment. The following vignettes illustrate the range of approaches required in outreach to adolescents who requested treatment during follow-up interviews.

Case Example: John—Hospitalized in Crisis

John, a 15-year-old Puerto Rican male, did not appear for initial appointments in the clinic; his case was thus closed, and he was randomly assigned to the monthly contact group. During the first follow-up call, John stated that he was depressed and had intermittent suicidal ideation without intent. The interviewer gave him the clinic number and suggested he call if he needed further information. Three days later John called, saying that, although ambivalent, he was interested in starting treatment. After assessing his suicide risk—John was currently depressed but without suicidal intent—the interviewer helped him create a list of potential positive and negative consequences of starting therapy, and began educating him about the process of therapy.

After this discussion, John decided he would like to try psychotherapy. The interviewer gave him referral information and prepared him for typical intake procedures. John wanted to make the call himself and did not want to involve his mother in the process. A verbal contract was made: John agreed that if he started to feel suicidal he would talk to a close friend, call the interviewer, or go directly to a local emergency room if necessary.

Eleven days later John called the interviewer, stating that he felt suicidal and needed help. He had called the community mental health center to which he was referred, but was never able to talk to anyone directly. After a brief assessment, the interviewer decided that John needed to go to the emergency room for an immediate evaluation; he did not resist this plan. The interviewer then told John that his mother needed to be informed. John's mother was angry at the interviewer for suggesting an emergency room evaluation because she felt her son was "just trying to get attention" and manipulate her. The interviewer empathized with her feelings of anger, helplessness, and worry, while emphasizing that the reason behind John's desire to die was not currently relevant; instead, the immediate goal was to ensure his safety, and an evaluation at the hospital was the most efficient way to do that. The mother eventually agreed to take him to the emergency room.

John was subsequently hospitalized; during his four-month stay in a psychiatric unit, the interviewer kept in contact, for supportive purposes, with John's mother. The mother was appreciative of this continued contact and expressed gratitude for the interviewer's assistance. At the fifth monthly call, John was home from the hospital and doing much better.

He had a scheduled appointment at a clinic later that week, which he planned to keep.

The next case illustrates both the difficulty in making a successful referral and the benefit of the monthly contacts.

Case Example: Jane—Treatment by Telephone

Jane, a 16-year-old Jamaican female, was not accepted for treatment in the clinic because of an apparent depression with psychotic features and suicidal ideation; she was referred directly to the emergency room and long-term treatment, and was randomly assigned to the monthly contact group. During the initial call, Jane stated that she felt depressed chronically and had intermittent suicidal ideation without intent. She was vague about whether she or her mother had scheduled any appointments for psychotherapy; she had not visited the emergency room. During this call, the interviewer also made contact with Jane's mother, giving her the same referral information Jane had been given and informing her of her daughter's intermittent suicidal ideation.

During the second monthly telephone call, Jane stated that she had not followed through with her scheduled appointment, but did not know why. The interviewer gave her the number of another mental health clinic, made a verbal suicide contract, and suggested she call back if she needed further assistance. One month later Jane was in much better spirits. The interviewer then talked to Jane's mother, who expressed concern about her daughter and wanted referral information to get her into treatment; she had lost the information previously given to her.

For the next several months, Jane and her mother did not follow through with referrals for various reasons. In the face of an apparently unorganized, perhaps even chaotic, household, Jane's mental state varied, from feeling depressed with suicidal ideation to more optimistic and not suicidal. Most notably, she became more talkative and engaged with the interviewer, stating that she recognized that she needed someone to talk to and that she could not rely on her mother to schedule an appointment for her. Because Jane continued to express suicidal ideation, however, the interviewer emphasized the importance of informing her mother about her current depression and the need for treatment. At the sixth month, Jane's mother had made an appointment at a clinic, for six weeks after the call.

The interviewer continued to maintain monthly contact with both Jane and her mother; Jane continued to make use of the telephone calls to express her feelings and concerns. Despite the fact that Jane and her mother did not keep the scheduled appointment for psychotherapy, Jane's mood appeared to lighten over the next three months. She became more engaged socially: She had made the school softball team, was getting better grades, and developed some friendships (including a boyfriend). When asked what had changed, Jane stated: "I had to take charge of my life and only I can do that." When the issue of treatment was raised, she stated that although she thought it would be helpful to talk with someone, she felt it was not currently necessary.

At the eleventh call, Jane continued to feel less depressed, denying suicidal ideation. The interviewer informed her that this would be her last contact, since the interviewer had taken a job in another state. Upon contact a month later by a different interviewer for her twelfth monthly call, Jane was again somewhat depressed and requested a referral for treatment. She was invited to apply for treatment in the clinic at which the interviewer was employed; one week later she appeared at the clinic for her initial evaluation session.

Clearly, this case raises the issue of the interviewer in the role of psychotherapist-by-telephone; this will be discussed further later. First, a third example describes an adolescent who was successfully readmitted into the clinic as a direct consequence of follow-up telephone contact.

Case Example: Ruth—Understanding the Process of Therapy

Ruth, a 15-year-old Dominican girl, was referred to the clinic initially after making a suicide attempt. At that time, she came to only a few sessions and then withdrew from treatment. During her first interview six months later, Ruth stated that she dropped out of treatment because she did not like attending sessions on a regular basis and wanted to talk with someone only when she felt like it; because this was not possible, she had decided to stop. Currently, things were better for her. Nevertheless, the interviewer invited her to call back if she decided she wanted to reenter treatment in the future.

One week later, Ruth called and stated that she thought over the telephone call and realized that she really did want someone to talk with about her problems. Because she dropped out of treatment initially, the interviewer spent time educating Ruth about the process of therapy and the need to come on a regular basis for treatment to be effective. Ruth agreed to make the necessary three-month commitment at the clinic; she was readmitted to the program and subsequently attended all sessions, deriving substantial benefit from treatment.

INTERVENTION AND OUTREACH

Each of these cases required different outreach interventions; the interviewer's role expanded to include crisis worker, case manager, and therapist. In the first vignette, John was ambivalent about starting treatment and used the follow-up contact to clarify his concerns. The influence of the PFPEP in bringing John into therapy was significant because initially he was noncompliant with treatment. The rapid establishment of an alliance enabled him to rely upon the interviewer as a support during his crisis. In the second case, Jane was interested in treatment, but her mother did not follow through with the referral. Therefore, the interviewer was compelled to play the role of both case manager and therapist. Near the end of the year, Jane revealed that she always anticipated the telephone calls, stating that they were helpful because they made her feel that someone cared about her. Interestingly, during contact after the interviewer (M.W.) left the clinic, Jane decided to begin face-to-face treatment; subsequently she was admitted to the clinic for psychotherapy and complied with scheduled appointments. This suggests quite clearly that the telephone contact was serving a psychotherapeutic function for her. Only further investigation would clarify whether telephone contact postponed face-to-face treatment or facilitated Jane's entry into the clinic itself.

In the third case, Ruth was brought back into treatment successfully as a result of follow-up contact, during which she was educated regarding the parameters of psychotherapy. Similar to the case of John, the interviewer worked with the adolescent on creating a list of the personal costs and benefits to starting treatment; this led to her decision to return to the clinic for further psychotherapy.

In all three cases, the adolescents were interested in treatment, albeit ambivalently; further, it is unlikely that contact with mental health services would have been initiated without benefit of the PFPEP. Both John and Ruth are examples of initial noncompliers with treatment. For them, the PFPEP provided a forum in which to discuss their concerns and become educated about the process of therapy. The case of Jane illustrates the difficulties encountered when parents are not compliant with the process of accessing treatment. Because she was not at imminent risk for suicide, social services could not be used as leverage. Without her mother's willingness to comply, successful follow-through became difficult, requiring the interviewer to function as a psychotherapist-by-telephone for nearly a year. The complexity of this case demonstrates the importance of building a working relationship with parents whenever possible when the clinician's goal is to bring an adolescent into treatment.

IMMINENT SUICIDAL RISK

Interaction with adolescents at imminent risk of suicidal behavior already has been discussed indirectly, but deserves further exploration. This section briefly describes the general protocol used when confronted with a suicidal crisis on the telephone; the description is followed by specific case examples.

When adolescents verbalized suicidal ideation during a PFPEP contact, further assessment was initiated immediately. If the adolescent was determined to be at current risk, the interviewer used a crisis-oriented approach and, if indicated, assisted in sending the adolescent to an emergency room in the following ways: First and typically, the option of hospitalization was discussed with both the adolescent and caregiver and a concrete plan was made over the telephone detailing how, with whom, and when the adolescent would go to the hospital. Second, the interviewer maintained contact until the adolescent arrived safely at the hospital and other professionals were involved actively. The following cases illustrate the variety of crises encountered during the PFPEP.

Case Example: Sue—Traumatized and Resistant

Sue, a 17-year-old Korean female who became actively suicidal after being raped, came for one appointment at the clinic and then decided not to return. She was randomly assigned to the monthly contact group. During the first call, Sue tentatively stated that she still felt depressed, but denied any suicidal ideation or intent. When asked if she wanted to reconsider treatment, she said she had thought about it; she was given referral information for the clinic and other area mental health services. At the second call, she was slightly more open with the interviewer, admitting to feeling depressed with occasional flashbacks of the rape; she also reported suicidal ideation without intent. The interviewer outlined the process of psychotherapy and how it might help her. Sue resisted having the interviewer talk to her parents, and this request was respected because she did not appear to be actively suicidal despite intermittent ideation.

By the third telephone call, Sue's depression and flashbacks had worsened; she also reported making two suicide attempts during the past month, having informed her mother about one of them. The attempts were overdoses of medication that did not necessitate hospitalization; nevertheless, both were serious in intent. Sue also refused to make a verbal contract over the telephone because she did not believe she could prevent herself from making suicide attempts in the near future. At that point, the interviewer insisted upon informing another family member of Sue's condition, since she refused to go to the hospital on her own. Since her parents were unable to be reached immediately, Sue's adult brother was contacted instead. He was ambivalent, but agreed to bring Sue to the emergency room that evening.

However, when the interviewer called to follow up on the intervention the next morning, Sue's brother stated that Sue had refused to go to the emergency room. The interviewer informed him that if the family did not bring Sue to the hospital that day, a mobile crisis team would be sent to their house to evaluate the situation and bring Sue to the hospital themselves if necessary. Sue's family then complied; she was subsequently hospitalized for two months, where she progressed significantly in treatment.

Case Example: Cindy—Crisis in Progress

Cindy, a 15-year-old black female, was referred to the clinic for depression and a history of a suicide attempt. Upon termination, she was randomly assigned to the monthly contact group. At the first month, the interviewer happened to call when Cindy and her father were in the midst of an argument. Cindy felt suicidal and thought she might need to go to the emergency room. Because of the suicide risk, the interviewer asked to speak with Cindy's father. The father expressed the belief that his daughter was not suicidal but was simply trying to manipulate him to get what she wanted. The interviewer spent about 45 minutes on the telephone with both Cindy and her father, helping them to understand each other's perspective so that some of the anger could be dissipated. By the end of the conversation, Cindy had stopped crying and denied any suicidal ideation or intent. The interviewer also reminded her father to observe Cindy closely and to bring her to the hospital if necessary. The interviewer also gave them information about a local community mental health clinic should they want to pursue treatment.

Each of these cases involved contact not only with the adolescent but with family members and various professionals. It is important to note that in the case of Sue, as well as John in the previous section, the nature of the crisis was not revealed during the initial monthly PFPEP contact. Only after an alliance was developed did the adolescents begin to speak more openly, asking for help and using the interviewer as a support. This speaks to the power of brief monthly contact with this high-risk population.

Moreover, PFPEP contacts, whether monthly or biannually, also allowed for immediate crisis intervention with adolescents and their families, as in the case of Cindy. The salient goal in such situations was to ensure the adolescent's safety and arrange appropriate treatment with other mental health professionals.

CONCLUSION

Although the initial intention of the PFPEP was to evaluate the effectiveness of treatment in the clinic and to assess the effect of a telephone follow-up procedure on recidivism, it quickly became clear that many adolescents contacted required immediate clinical intervention for acute conditions. By describing the different categories of outreach that have been implemented through the PFPEP, it is hoped that other researchers and clinicians will systematically study and expand upon the use of telephone follow-up with suicidal adolescents.

Like Tausig and Freeman (1988) and Reich and Earls (1990), we found the telephone to be an effective medium through which to contact adolescents and their families. Most of the participating adolescents and parents stated that they found telephone contact useful as well. In the words of one adolescent: "I like the fact that you keep in touch. It's nice to know that if I get upset about something in the future, I can call." A number of adolescents stated that it felt good to know that there was someone who cared about them. Caregivers often described the interviewer as an "ally"; perhaps the most poignant comment came from John's mother, who thanked the interviewer for "saving my son's life." Clearly, among individuals and families whose resources and supports are limited, the knowledge that a concerned professional is available can be at least salutory, if not frankly therapeutic.

Finally, many adolescents continue to be at risk for suicide after a suicide attempt, as is well documented in the literature (Davidson & Linnoila, 1989; Holinger, 1989; Pfeffer, 1989; Pfeffer et al., 1991; Pfeffer et al., 1993; Spirito, 1990; Spirito et al., 1989; Spirito et al., 1991). Although many adolescents are noncompliant with mental health treatment, some apparently not only still need services, but want further treatment; the PFPEP contact provided one way to assist these individuals in accessing the services they still needed. The program also allowed direct and focal access to at-risk adolescents, as recommended by Shaffer and his colleagues (Shaffer et al., 1990; Shaffer et al., 1991).

Logically, one is pressed to consider why such adolescents are noncompliant with treatment recommendations despite recognizing themselves that they need and desire help. Some hypotheses, from a number of vantage points, can be drawn from the clinical material gathered through the PFPEP. First, from a systems perspective, one obvious hindrance is the actual difficulty involved in scheduling appointments and being seen for psychotherapy at community mental health centers. Currently, most publicly funded mental health clinics in the inner-city neighborhoods in which the PFPEP was implemented have two- to three-month waiting lists; frequently, adolescents cannot tolerate the frustration of such a waiting period. Consequently, the PFPEP interviewer attempted to "inoculate" the adolescents and their families so that they could anticipate the arduous process of gaining access to treatment.

Second, ambivalence was a recurrent theme for adolescents in the PFPEP who inquired about further treatment. Many had stereotypic views about psychotherapy, anticipating shame and fearing social approbation. Frequently, adolescents as well as their parents also feared that if they delved into their problems, they might become more suicidal rather than attenuating those self-destructive impulses. In response to these concerns, the interviewer educated participants about the process and benefits of psychotherapy, directly addressing the resistances to initiating the process.

Third, and certainly not surprisingly, parental involvement was found to be another important factor in treatment compliance. Many parents discussed feeling overwhelmed and helpless, experiencing themselves as "bad parents." Telephone contact was a forum for many of them to receive support and clarify the available options in helping their children.

It is undoubtedly apparent that further research is needed to determine more definitively whether telephone interventions actually decrease the risk of suicide in high-risk adolescent populations. Among other issues, the work described here does not inform us what are the long-term consequences of telephone interventions. Nevertheless, the clinical vignettes described in this chapter suggest strongly that the short-term impact is positive in many cases and that frequency and timeliness of contact may have increased compliance. In fact, several young lives may well have been saved by timely and consistent intervention by telephone.

REFERENCES

Chambers, W. J., Puig-Antich, J., Hirsch, M., Paez, P., Ambrosini, P. J., Tabrizi, M. A., & Davies, M. (1985). The assessment of affective disorders in children and adolescents by semistructured interview. *Archives of General Psychiatry, 42*, 697–702.

Clarke, C. F. (1988). Deliberate self-poisoning in adolescents. *Archives of the Disturbed Child, 63*(12), 1479–1483.

Davidson, L., & Linnoila, M. (Eds.) (1989). *Report of the secretary's task force on youth suicide: (Vol. 2). Risk factors for youth suicide.* DHHS Pub. No. (ADM) 89-1622. Washington, DC: U.S. Government Printing Office.

Frankel, B. S., & Hovell, M. F. (1978). Health service appointment keeping: A behavioral view and critical review. *Behavior Modification, 2*(4), 435–464.

Hengeveld, M. W., van Egmond, M., Bouwmans, P. M., & van Rooyen, L. (1991). Suicide risk in female suicide attempters not responding to a follow-up study. *Acta Pscyhiatrica Scandinavia, 83*, 142–144.

Holinger, P. C. (1989). Epidemiological issues in youth suicide. In C. R. Pfeffer (Ed.), *Suicide among youth: Perspectives on risk and prevention* (pp. 41–62). Washington, DC: American Psychiatric Press.

Litt, I. F., Cuskey, W. R., & Rudd, S. (1983). Emergency room evaluation of the adolescent who attempts suicide: Compliance with follow-up. *Journal of Adolescent Health Care, 4*, 106–108.

Nardini-Maillard, D., & Ladame, F. G. (1980). The results of a follow-up study of suicidal adolescents. *Journal of Adolescence, 3,* 253–260.

Paulsen, A. S., Crowe, R. R., Noyes, R., & Pfohl, B. (1988). Reliability of the telephone interview in diagnosing anxiety disorders. *Archives of General Psychiatry, 45,* 62–63.

Pfeffer, C. R. (1989). Life stress and family risk factors for youth fatal and nonfatal suicidal behavior. In C. R. Pfeffer (Ed.), *Suicide among youth: Perspectives on risk and prevention* (pp. 143–164). Washington, DC: American Psychiatric Press.

Pfeffer, C. R., Klerman, G. L., Hurt, S. W., Kakuna, T., Peskin, J. R., & Siefker, C. A. (1993). Suicidal children grow up: Rates and psychosocial risk factors for suicide attempts during follow-up. *Journal of the American Academy of Child and Adolescent Psychiatry, 32*(1), 106–113.

Pfeffer, C. R., Klerman, G. L., Hurt, S. W., Lesser, M., Peskin, J. R., & Siefker, C. A. (1991). Suicidal children grow up: Demographic and clinical risk factors for adolescent suicide attempts. *Journal of the American Academy of Child and Adolescent Psychiatry, 30*(4), 609–616.

Pfeffer, C. R., Peskin, J. R., & Siefker, C. A. (1992). Suicidal children grow up: Psychiatric treatment during follow-up period. *Journal of the American Academy of Child and Adolescent Psychiatry, 31*(4), 679–685.

Reich, W., & Earls, F. (1990). Interviewing adolescents by telephone: Is it a useful methodological strategy? *Comprehensive Psychiatry, 31*(3), 211–215.

Rotheram, M. J. (1990, October). *The treatment of adolescents who have attempted suicide.* Institute presentation at the 37th Annual Meeting of the American Academy of Child and Adolescent Psychiatry, Chicago, IL.

Shaffer, D., Garland, A., Vieland, V., Whittle, B., Underwood, M., & Busner, C. (1991). The impact of curriculum-based suicide prevention programs. *Journal of the American Academy of Child and Adolescent Psychiatry, 30*(4), 588–596.

Shaffer, D., Vieland, V., Garland, A., Rojas, M., Underwood, M., & Busner, C. (1990). Adolescent suicide attempters: Response to suicide prevention programs. *Journal of the American Medical Association, 264,* 3151–3155.

Spirito, A. (1990, October). *Follow-up studies of adolescent suicide attempters.* Materials prepared for the 37th Annual Meeting of the American Academy of Child and Adolescent Psychiatry. Chicago, IL.

Spirito, A., Brown, L., Overholser, J., & Fritz, G. (1989). Attempted suicide in adolescence: A review and critique of the literature. *Clinical Psychology Review, 9,* 335–363.

Spirito, A., Plummer, B., Gispert, M., Levy, S., Kurkjian, J., Lewander, W., Hagberg, S., & Devost, L. (1992). Adolescent suicide attempts: Outcomes at follow-up. *American Journal of Orthopsychiatry, 62*(3), 464–468.

Tausig, J. E., & Freeman, E. W. (1988). The next best thing to being there: Conducting the clinical research interview by telephone. *American Journal of Orthopsychiatry, 58*(3), 418–427.

Trautman, P. D., & Rotheram, M. J. (1986, October). *Referral failure among adolescent suicide attempters.* Poster presented at the 33rd Annual Meeting of the American Academy of Child Psychiatry, Los Angeles, CA.

Trautman, P. D., & Stewart, N. (1989, October). *Are adolescent suicide attempters non-compliant with outpatient care?* Poster presented at the 36th Annual Meeting of the American Academy of Child Psychiatry, New York.

Vieland, V., Whittle, B., Garland, A., Hicks, R., & Shaffer, D. (1991). The impact of curriculum-based suicide prevention programs for teenagers: An 18-month follow-up. *Journal of the American Academy of Child and Adolescent Psychiatry, 30*(5), 811–815.

Zimmerman, J. K., & Woodard, M. G. (1993, April). *Long-term follow-up with suicidal adolescents: Description and preliminary findings.* Paper presented at the 26th Annual Conference of the American Association of Suicidology, San Francisco, CA.

PART IV
Conclusion

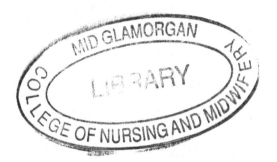

14

Summary and Future Directions

JAMES K. ZIMMERMAN

In Chapter 1 of this volume, I considered the value and possible efficacy of treating suicidal adolescents. Initially I asked whether such treatment works, and whether it is "worth it" for the mental health professional. In the ensuing chapters, a number of authors have presented various approaches designed to address this issue from a clinical perspective; clearly, there is a strong feeling among them that their work is not for naught and that it is worthwhile. It is hoped that the reader has gained some insight into both the methods employed with suicidal adolescents and the experience one might expect to have in the process.

In this closing chapter, I would like to revisit the questions raised in the first chapter of this volume: Does treatment with suicidal adolescents actually work? Is it worth the undertaking? Following that, I discuss briefly a method to determine which approach to treatment might be most likely to lead to a positive therapeutic outcome in a given case. Finally, I consider pathways toward enhancing our understanding of the treatment of suicidal adolescents in the future.

DOES IT REALLY WORK?

Despite the depth of investigation represented in the chapters of this volume, the question of treatment efficacy with suicidal adolescents must remain answerable only in somewhat ambiguous terms. The most positive answer that can be given is a yes, sometimes. Clearly, there are cases presented herein and elsewhere (e.g., Berman & Jobes, 1991; Fishman, 1988) that give evidence of successful treatment, accompanied by waning or cessation of suicidality and improved psychosocial functioning; nevertheless, there is the research—also presented in Chapter 1 of this volume—that raises concerns about long-term outcomes for suicidal adolescents regardless of the amount and type of treatment they have received (Feiner, Adan, & Silverman, 1992; Muehrer, 1990; Pfeffer et al., 1994; Pfeffer, Peskin, & Siefker, 1992).

Moreover, even within the context of clinical studies, it is evident that improvement does not always occur in a linear, positive trajectory. Movement toward psychological health and (it is hoped) optimal functioning is not an easy process for suicidal teens; in fact, it is often fraught with setbacks, resurgences of suicidality, and painful or even harrowing interpersonal and environmental circumstances that militate against it. Thus, despite apparently clear-cut and well-documented success stories from the clinical case study literature, the question of treatment efficacy, particularly over the longer term, must remain only provisionally and tentatively answered: Yes, those who treat suicidal adolescents believe it works, at least in some cases and to some extent.

IS IT REALLY WORTH IT?

Is the treatment of suicidal adolescents worth the effort, given the preceding questions about its efficacy, along with the toll it takes in stress on the practitioner involved? The answer to this question may be somewhat simpler than that to the question of treatment efficacy, although the answer still is unlikely to be a resounding, "Yes, of course!"

The debatable point here, the mitigating circumstance, is more a personal, individual one that must be pondered by any mental health professional faced with the possibility of developing a practice, or working in a clinical setting, that includes suicidal adolescents. Rather than whether it is "really worth it," the real question is this: Can I manage the stress, can I titrate the anxiety and self-doubt, can I metabolize the countertransference, so that I can be effective in treating these patients? As was described in Chapter 1, and brought to life and enriched by subsequent chapters in this book, clinicians must take a certain stance in order to treat suicidal adolescents. Those who can do so often find the work immensely rewarding; perhaps others should not engage in such practice at all, or should do so only as a very minor component of their total caseload and with strong support from colleagues or supervisors. (See, for example, Richman, 1986.)

The choice to commit a portion of one's practice to suicidal adolescents is one that can be made clearly only through an introspective search. Even at that, it is a decision that ought to be reviewed periodically to determine if it is still valid and practicable.

SELECTION OF TREATMENT APPROACH

In the chapters of this book, the authors have presented a number of different approaches to intervention, based on various, and perhaps sometimes divergent, theoretical and technical perspectives. Although enlightening, this cluster of viewpoints also may lead to a certain level of confusion regarding clinical intervention. Simply put, given that one has decided that treating suicidal adolescents is worthwhile and worth it, how is the decision made regarding the intervention to be offered in any specific case? Is it possible to make a lucid, well-informed choice about treatment selection, given the many variables with which one is presented in this undertaking?

The concept of treatment selection based on a systematized method is an issue being considered seriously and intensively in the current mental health environment. (See, for example, Beutler and Clarkin, 1990.) The fundamental idea, perhaps the hope, is that each symptom picture, each presenting case could dictate definitively the ensuing treatment approach. In actual practice, however, this is not an easy decision to make. Often one's approach to treatment is structured by the setting in which treatment is offered or is constrained by the unwillingness of some patients or family members to participate. Further, one's own training, experience, and comfort level in adopting a given strategy must be taken into account as well.

Although a full consideration of this question is worthy of many volumes, I would like to suggest a general approach, taking into account several components, which may allow for a decision to be made regarding treatment selection. This approach is pragmatic, employing the features of the presenting case as the starting point, rather than cleaving to a preconceived conceptualization of what suicidal adolescents should be offered generically in treatment. Ideally, the approach to intervention will arise organically from the needs of the patient and the available points of access to his or her world. Components, each to be discussed briefly, include the following: adolescent's symptom presentation and diagnosis; family's symptom presentation; leverage points;

integrative approaches; and ability to engage and keep the patient(s) in treatment.

Symptoms and Diagnosis

Although it may seem self-evident that treatment should be shaped by the symptoms and diagnosis of the patient, this is worth emphasizing here. The risk is in taking too simplistic an approach to intervention, either by assuming that all suicidal adolescents need similar treatment *because* they are suicidal, or by assuming that all individuals with a given diagnosis warrant the same approach without taking into consideration the subtleties of their particular symptom presentation. It is rather easy to convince a suicidal adolescent not to return for further treatment by either ignoring or overemphasizing his or her suicidality; likewise, treatment is unlikely to be successful if other diagnostic factors—such as depressive symptoms, post-traumatic stress disorder, history of sexual or physical abuse, and so on—are not taken into account. A thorough but balanced initial interview and assessment is essential to the success of treatment.

Family Symptomatology

When an adolescent is suicidal, frequently the etiology is at least partially to be discovered in the family system. Similarly, as family dynamics impinge on the adolescent, so does the adolescent's behavior affect family functioning. Here again, the likely error is in taking too narrow a focus, so that one treats the adolescent and does not take into account factors in the family that engender suicidal behavior in the teenager. One can then keep the treatment pure and elegant, and perhaps contain one's own anxiety more effectively, while losing the patient entirely in the process. Additionally, possible supportive or ameliorative potentials in the family will be left in the detritus of a failed intervention. In fact, some suicidologists believe that it is nonsensical to treat a suicidal adolescent without intervening with the family as well (Brent, 1994; Richman, 1986). As is the case with the adolescent, a systemic assessment of sufficient breadth and depth is vital to effective intervention.

Leverage Points

When one is confronted with a suicidal adolescent as a possible psychotherapy patient, there are a number of different facets to the issues with which one is faced. These facets can provide several avenues of entry into the adolescent's life, or what I consider to be *leverage points* in treatment. Gustafson (1986), referring to these as positions or levels of observation, suggested that one must enter where one can and be prepared to shift one's level of observation (and therefore, one's leverage points for intervention) when necessary.

Leverage points can be found within the individual, in the family system, or in larger social systems, such as the school or the child welfare system. For example, if an adolescent, unwilling to discuss his or her suicide attempt at the outset, is willing nevertheless to enter into treatment, the initial phase of intervention can focus on other areas of concern, such as the adolescent's relationships with peers or performance in school. This intrapersonal shift of leverage point may lead the adolescent to feel more comfortable engaging in treatment; the issue of suicidality can be returned to at a later time. On the other hand, if an adolescent is preoccupied with suicidal thoughts and is unable to consider methods for attenuating the intensity of the ideation, then perhaps the introduction of other family members into treatment would be necessary. This shift in point of leverage from the individual to the family system may allow for protective factors, such as family support and concern, to be employed.

The introduction of larger social systems as leverage points in treating suicidal adolescents takes the clinician into other realms, such as case management. This can be quite useful in some instances, and one may be compelled to involve social systems in others. For example, if one suspects that a substrate of the adolescent's suicidality may be a learning disability, it would be salient to be in contact with the school. This contact would be implemented to determine the exact nature of problems in learning, to inform the school of such problems if one had done the assessment, or to assist the school in developing an educational program appropriate for the adolescent's needs. In some cases, assistance in ameliorating the adolescent's academic problems can be a major component in reducing his or her suicidality. (See, for example, Zimmerman, 1994.)

The involvement of the child welfare system is a step that many clinicians resist, despite their awareness of its legal necessity when abuse or neglected is identified or suspected. Nevertheless, there are times when this is the only apparent leverage point with which one is left, such as when an adolescent is actively suicidal and the family is unorganized enough or resistant enough that intervention is not possible. In such cases, the participation of the child welfare system (and agencies such as mobile crisis teams where available) can be the gateway to helping the adolescent access mental health services, even if such services are provided in a hospital emergency room or through involuntary placement in a psychiatric institution.

In sum, then, an approach that considers carefully what are the available leverage points, and which point of entry into the world of the adolescent is likely to be most productive at any given time, can help enhance the likelihood that treatment ultimately will be effective.

Integrative Approaches

In light of this, it probably is clear that the most profitable leverage point may shift during the treatment process, perhaps even several times. In order to implement interventions that take into account various leverage points and their transformations, an integrative approach to treatment is likely to be necessary. Technical combinations of psychodynamic, cognitive-behavioral, and family systems approaches may be useful; so might combinations of modalities, such as individual, family, and group psychotherapy in the optimal treatment of one individual. Moreover, interventions that integrate the facilities of several larger systems, such as the private therapy office, the school, and the psychiatric emergency room, may be necessary.

Such an approach to the implementation of treatment requires a certain flexibility and ability to shift stances on the part of the clinician. It should be quite apparent that such a posture is predicated upon exposure to and comfort with a number of different conceptualizations of treatment, along with a familiarity with a range of technical approaches. Clearly, then, to adopt this view of treatment, and to implement it, has consequences for the education and training of clinicians; such issues are beyond what can be discussed here. Suffice it to say that, in treating suicidal adolescents, breadth as well as depth of experience and training are vital in providing the best interventions one can. In some cases, success in treatment may depend on one's flexibility and comfort with textural complexity; in addition, one's ability to shift stances rapidly in response to the demands of the situation can be substantially important.

Engaging and Keeping Suicidal
Adolescents in Treatment

It is one thing to engage suicidal adolescents initially in the treatment process; clinical experience and research evidence both can attest to the fact that that is difficult enough (Clarke, 1988; Rotheram-Borus, 1990; Swedo, 1989; Trautman & Rotheram, 1986). It is perhaps even a greater challenge to keep them in treatment once they are there. Much has been written about the attributes of clinicians, and the characteristics of patient-therapist relationships, that are likely to lead to successful treatment (e.g., Beutler & Clarkin, 1990); anything but a brief consideration of this subject is beyond the scope of this chapter. However, it can be said that one might be compelled to tailor one's style to the needs of a suicidal adolescent and his or her family in order to enhance the likelihood that treatment will begin, continue, and arrive at a satisfactory conclusion. As mentioned earlier, flexibility in one's technical approach often is called for; likewise, a more relaxed and perhaps even self-revealing stance frequently is required.

In addition, given the crisis-oriented nature of much intervention with suicidal adolescents, a somewhat more directive, and certainly more active, approach is likely to be necessary. Further, resistances and misunderstandings need immediate confrontation, since treatment may otherwise end abruptly with the patient's withdrawal; with adolescents in a suicidal crisis, there is seldom the luxury of allowing the working alliance and transference to develop and ripen at a leisurely pace.

FIVE COMPONENTS REVISITED

In sum, then, the approach to treating suicidal adolescents presented here requires thorough and intensive initial assessment interviews of both the adolescent and significant family members. This is essential not only to arrive at some sense of what symptoms need addressing and what diagnostic areas one might need to be cognizant of, but also to obtain an understanding of what leverage points are most likely to bear therapeutic fruit within a short period of time. Given this perspective on the case, one then proceeds in a manner that is direct, immediate, and flexible. This approach allows for shifts in the stage on which treatment occurs, not only technically, but also with regard to the modalities and systems through which it is delivered.

FUTURE DIRECTIONS

The future of adolescent suicidology is complex, and is likely to require thrusts in a number of directions if clarity is to be achieved in understanding the etiology of adolescent suicide as well as effective techniques of intervention and prevention. Impressive empirical and clinical research has been done in the areas of etiology (e.g., Lester, 1992; Pfeffer, 1989), assessment and prediction (e.g., Maris, Berman, Maltsberger, & Yufit, 1992), intervention (e.g., Berman & Jobes, 1991), and prevention (e.g., Leenaars & Wenckstern, 1991). It is vital that such work continue. Moreover, long-term follow-up research (e.g., Paarregaard, 1975; Pfeffer, Peskin, & Siefker, 1992; Pfeffer et al., 1994) is essential to understand more definitively what can be implemented that is effective in reducing recidivism, as are controlled treatment outcome studies. The latter are not yet available, and would be necessary to further delineate the value of various forms of clinical intervention.

Finally, advances in the understanding of suicidality in adolescence and its treatment and prevention will be most enhanced by a cross-pollination between clinicians and researchers, such that clinicians are well informed regarding the findings of research and researchers are sensitized to the experience of clinicians who are providing front-line intervention. Without such interaction and collaboration on a consistent basis, qualitative clinical insight and quantitative empirical understanding would exist in parallel, nonintersecting universes. This would be a great loss to both, since each perspective has much to offer to the other in depth and breadth of knowledge. Sadly, the ultimate victims would be the very individuals—suicidal adolescents—whose pain we are all attempting to alleviate, perhaps even whose lives we are striving to save.

REFERENCES

Berman, A. L., & Jobes, D. A. (1991). *Adolescent suicide: Assessment and intervention.* Washington, DC: American Psychological Association.

Beutler, L. E., & Clarkin, J. F. (1990). *Systematic treatment selection: Toward targeted therapeutic interventions.* New York: Brunner/Mazel.

Brent, D. (1994, April). *Reducing the toll: Youth suicide prevention.* Theme address at the 27th Annual Meeting of the American Association of Suicidology, New York.

Clarke, C. F. (1988). Deliberate self-poisoning in adolescents. *Archives of Disorders of Childhood, 63,* 1479–1483.

Feiner, R. D., Adan, A. M., & Silverman, M. M. (1992). Risk assessment and prevention of youth suicide in schools and educational contexts. In R. W. Maris, A. L. Berman, J. T. Maltsberger, & R. I. Yufit (Eds.), *Assessment and prediction of suicide* (pp. 420–447). New York: The Guilford Press.

Fishman, H. C. (1988). *Treating troubled adolescents: A family therapy approach.* New York: Basic Books.

Gustafson, J. P. (1986). *The complex secret of brief psychotherapy.* New York: W.W. Norton.

Leenaars, A. A., & Wenckstern, S. (1991). *Suicide prevention in schools.* New York: Hemisphere Publishing.

Lester, D. (1992). *Why people kill themselves* (3rd ed.). Springfield, IL: Charles C. Thomas.

Maris, R. W., Berman, A. L., Maltsberger, J. T., & Yufit, R. I. (Eds.) (1992). *Assessment and prediction of suicide.* New York: The Guilford Press.

Muehrer, P. (1990). *Conceptual research models for preventing mental disorders* (DHHS Publications No. ADM 90-1713). Rockville, MD: National Institute of Mental Health.

Paarregaard, G. (1975). Suicide among attempted suicides: A 10-year follow-up. *Suicide and Life-Threatening Behavior, 5*(3), 140–144.

Pfeffer, C. R. (1989). Life stress and family risk factors for youth fatal and nonfatal suicidal behavior. In C. R. Pfeffer (Ed.), *Suicide among youth: Perspectives on risk and prevention* (pp. 143–164). Washington, DC: American Psychiatric Press.

Pfeffer, C. R., Hurt, S. W., Kakuma, T., Peskin, J. R., Siefker, C. A., & Nagabhairava, S. (1994). Suicidal children grow up: Suicidal episodes and effects of treatment during follow-up. *Journal of the American Academy of Child and Adolescent Psychiatry, 33,* 225–230.

Pfeffer, C. R., Peskin, J. R., & Siefker, C. A. (1992). Suicidal children grow up: Psychiatric treatment during follow-up period. *Journal of the American Academy of Child and Adolescent Psychiatry, 31*(4), 679–685.

Richman, J. (1986). *Family therapy for suicidal people.* New York: Springer Publishing.

Rotheram-Borus, M. J. (1990, October). *The treatment of adolescents who have attempted suicide.* Institute presentation at the Annual Meeting of the American Academy of Child and Adolescent Psychiatry, Chicago, IL.

Swedo, S. E. (1989). Postdischarge therapy of hospitalized adolescent suicide attempters. *Journal of Adolescent Health Care, 10,* 541–544.

Trautman, P. D., & Rotheram, M. J. (1986, October). *Referral failure among adolescent suicide attempters.* Poster presented at the Annual Meeting of the American Academy of Child Psychiatry, Los Angeles, CA.

Zimmerman, J. K. (1994, April). *The do-gooder with two faces: The case of a 17-year-old male suicide attempter.* Paper presented at the 27th Annual Meeting of the American Association of Suicidology, New York.

Author Index

277

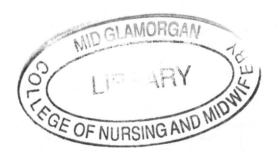

Subject Index